Aged Urine

Re-

Discovery Of

The Century

Dedicated to al l the open minded and those considering practicing the mightiest of all health protocols, and to those who already practice who seek more info!

Whether Your Mind Lies Close To The Earth

Or Whether It Soars To The Skies

You Will Find In This Book Exactly The Worth

That You Place On How High You Would Rise

If The Effort To Climb Is Too Great Or Severe

To Achieve A Goal That's Worth While,

You Might Better Stop *Reading* This Book Now,

And Grow Old In The Old Fashioned Style.

To You Who Are Ready To Fight For Change

From A Tired And Sluggish Existence,

This Complete Reversal Will Not Seem Too Strange

To Try Out For A While, With Persistance

Other Books By This Author

-Aged Urine: Discovery Of The Century

-Sunlight And Sungazing:- The Healing Power Of The Sun Ancient Knowledge For Modern Times

-Negative Ions: The Grand Unifier Of Health And Life

-This Meditation Will Transform Your Life: The Power Of Transcendental Meditation

Testimonials

"Your first book on Aged Urine changed my life. I had been ageing my urine for a year before stumbling upon it on Amazon but I didn't have the balls to drink the aged urine until I read your 6 and I had never thought about holding the aged urine for an extended period of time. That practice alone has had the BIGGEST impact on my experience. The results are not as instantaneous as drinking it but I've been doing it consistently for a week now and a couple of things have been happening. 1)my intuition has gone through the roof.2)I can physically see the spirits, angels, and guides now. It's something I've been working on for a couple of years, and I was able to see flashes of light before when they were present but now their presence is OBVIOUS and undeniable like another person standing in the room in the room with me.3)My life and dream realities are beginning to blur together. It's hard to explain but it's like the 3D and 4D are blended together which happened to me previously but rarely. Like a dream dejavu throughout the day if that makes any sense! Anyway, so grateful for your message and content."- Jennifer Ann

"I feel blissed out after ingesting aged urine for sure. Aged Urine affects my mood and energy more quickly than fresh and instantaneously makes me feel better and higher vibrations" -Jennifer Ann

Urine therapy has been a game changer for sure. UT has in and of itself been profound but the aged stuff brings it to a whole new level. Snorting, drinking and rubbing it on my skin has an immediate effect the brightens my whole system. Seeing this I started working on increasing my collection. Now have jars all over the place It blows my mind that this water of life is freely available and custom made for us. We have a tap of our own medicine that helps to increase our vibration and cleanse us out. Slowly rediscovering that we are truly free energy generators." -Vimal

Speaking on my aged urine book

"I read the book yesterday, even though I did quite some with urine lately (like making it most of my daily fluid intake since august this year), I used aged urine only sparingly. the book has been game changer, I started to rub it, use in ears, and ordered some canisters for storage, some spray bottles, eye droppers, an enema bulb and such, and will progressively integrate this approach. also started drinking aged urine in the morning, feels good, so far, I only did morning urine, as well as what I collected over night.

*O*ther ways of how I use it not mentioned in the book: swishing, eyebathing (in this case using an eye bathtub, yet will do the spraying thing, too), as well as adding quite some aged urine to bathwater, like 2 liters (not sure how effective this is). thanks again, I feel like this is a gem right in front of the worlds face, and almost nobody making use of it. I have a great feeling about this, also it seems very natural to do. and my body loves it. eager to go deeper into this- Michael Tmbltr

Aged urine ✦ORIN✦ is the most powerful elixir in existence, this ◉ am 100% certain of. Eye am on day 3 of a dry fast with the exception of a full wine glass of my 6month aged Orin. Nothing compares to this. Eye do no breathwork, my highly oxygenated orin does it all for me. Why work when you can play. This is the easiest dry fasting Eye have ever done in my life only because of this powerful blood plasma. That's what your urine is> your sacred blood plasma. Eye don't drink for the taste, Eye drink for the powerful cleaning and accelerated purification of my body. The only way out is in !

This is the plasma reset. And it's not happening out there it's happening inside of you...inside of us.

The moment it goes down my throat my whole body tingles, it electrifies....similar to the feeling when you take drugs. Then Eye see all the hairs on my body stand up like goosebumps but Eye am not cold at all. Eye put my hand to my heart and my heart is beating so fast. An overwhelming sense of peace, clarity, ECSTASY washes over me. Similar to drugs but millions n millions times better. Eye used to take a lot of chemical drugs for a very long time.

Eye now know this is the feeling Eye was seeking. Deep inside me Eye knew that this feeling of supreme ecstasy was my natural state. Except eye never needed the drugs it's been inside me all along... Eye only needed to purify and clean my temple. Aged orin is the bridge that got me here✦

Sure it doesn't taste pleasant but neither does blue cheese, parmesan, or even a lot of alcoholic spirits but Eye used to gauge on all of them in the past imagining it was some delicacy and caused so much harm and destruction to my cells. Aged orin does not cause any harm, only deep healing, it enables purification of the temple and a complete opening of all the chakras. Eye have never experienced anything like it. If you have tried wormwood herb or even dr Sebi bromide powder (seamoss) well aged orin is no where near as pungent as either of these ....there's so much more to tell but Eye am too high to be typing on this screen.

Eye love you and so eye share this sacred and ancient knowledge from my heart to yours to inspire you on your journey to a constant state of bliss. Please follow my wonderful sister @monicashuett in her stories right now is the most beautiful synchronisation of her knowledge about aged urine therapy crafted into digital he(ART)work. She has been drinking and using her orin for over 20 years and she is my greatest inspiration and dearest teacher. Eye am eternally greatful to Monica and my only desire is to inspire you in the same way that she inspired me. if this resonates she also has a YouTube Chanel with so many videos full of wisdom. There is nothing to buy here, nothing to sell ...only a knowledge and a gift from God that is inside of you. We are the ones we have been waiting for ...so why wait..? -Jes Sie

"Aged Urine: It ages so we don't have to." -Carlos Garcia

Harry Matadeen Yes absolutely! Sun bathing, sun gazing, UT, solarized rain water, breathing exercises, meditation. I'm in a good place today! There's a lot of things I did today because of you! Thank you so much for sharing so many beneficial life habits. Full of energy, happy and grateful!

-Prana Mellisha

Hi Harry Matadeen and your connections on FB that are still feeling resistance towards UT (not ready to post this on my own timeline... yet)

Here is my update on UT. After huge initial resistance I kept being drawn to it. Aged two bottles that are now 4 months+ and suninfused. Started with some fresh drops in eyes, on skin (little injuries, itchy spots, mosquito bites) and in homeopathic doses orally to conquer my aversion and was convinced by its medicinal qualities immediately.

Since two weeks I am looping fresh urine consistently and the taste is absolutely amazing: sweet and neutral, the more clean I eat (...fruits), the better it tastes). I am amazed!

The spiritual/energetic effects just blow me away: It is like in the movie Avatar where the beings plug in the tree of life with their hair. It is like putting the plug in my own socket. It is an absolutely intimate and familiar act of drinking my water of life, of drinking myself, Anke.

Also on the physical level I am experiencing great benefits: biggest one is that it stops any cravings for food. I am simply not hungry nor craving for junk. What a liberation!

Second effect is that I have an energetic and physical blockage in my stomach/small intestine for 20 years that I havent been able to cure yet, that put me on the path of cleaning up my diet. As soon as the urine passes that painful spot it starts to loosen up and the energy there gets into motion.

Third effect is that it helps with regular bowel movements. Enemas are my friend, but I feel I am not dependent on them anymore!

I am excited about this. Another ↤ to raising my vibration and taking my well being to a next level. I am currently in Italy visiting the pranic festival and look forward coming home and start the aged. No resistance left, just multiplied pure JOY.

Thank you for you exposing yourself and what you believe in so shamelessly to the world. I definetely received a ♦ here. Priceless 🖤

Anke

"Hi Harry. You could never wear me down from Urine therapy or any other health protocols that you happen to stumble upon. One of the many reasons I prefer to watch, even re-watch your videos, over watching many other Youtuber's videos would be due to how passionate you are and an almost endless source of some of the most valuable informationover a short course of time.

I hadn't thought about it until I watched your video. I allow my german shephard to sleep in my bed, when he does he tends to curl up and rest his head around my calves. Which in turn, causes me to lay still. In that proccess I've noticed a massive warmth creep on me throughout my body. For years I wondered why. Honestly thanks man, for always leaving me wanting to watch more content you provide or dig furtherin understanding these protocols.

I highly respect, appreciate and applaud you for the time you've invested into sharing your knowledge, experiences, and how its manifested your journey. Finding your channel and viewing the content has never been a waste of time. Again, thanks brother. Cheers"

-Dominic rivera.

Fresh Urine

This being the sequel to my first book on aged urine, (the first ever too

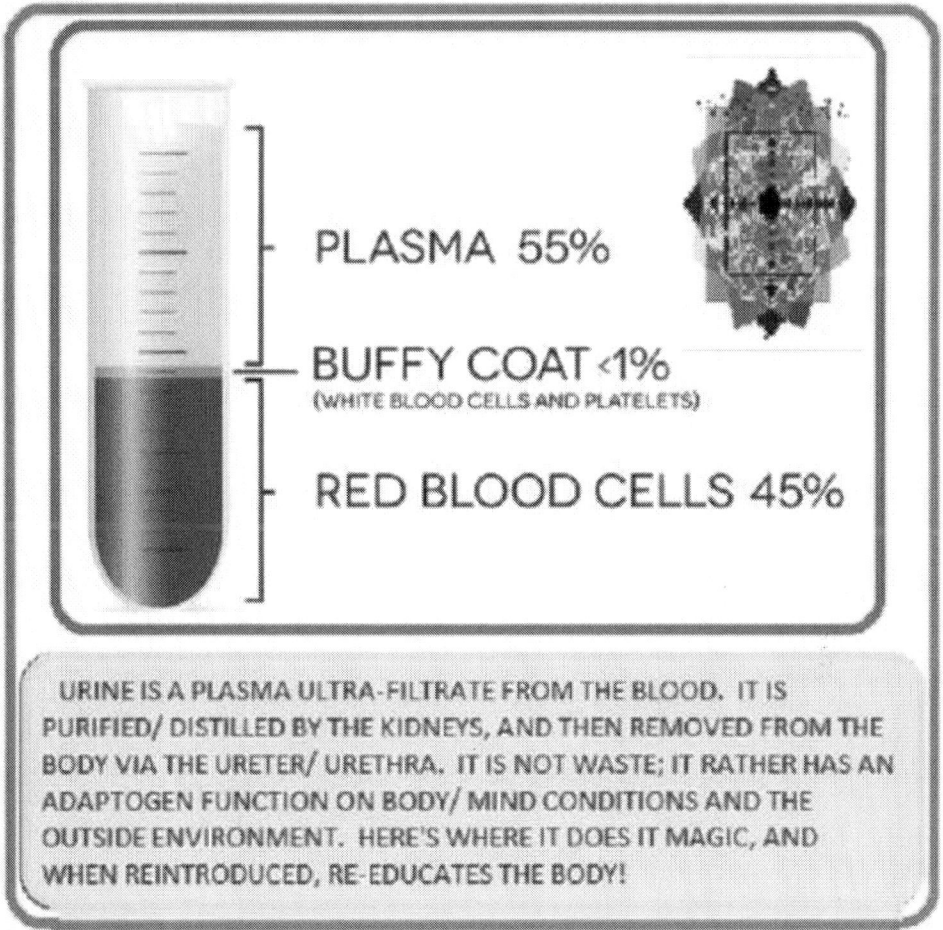

PLASMA 55%

BUFFY COAT <1%
(WHITE BLOOD CELLS AND PLATELETS)

RED BLOOD CELLS 45%

URINE IS A PLASMA ULTRA-FILTRATE FROM THE BLOOD. IT IS PURIFIED/ DISTILLED BY THE KIDNEYS, AND THEN REMOVED FROM THE BODY VIA THE URETER/ URETHRA. IT IS NOT WASTE; IT RATHER HAS AN ADAPTOGEN FUNCTION ON BODY/ MIND CONDITIONS AND THE OUTSIDE ENVIRONMENT. HERE'S WHERE IT DOES IT MAGIC, AND WHEN REINTRODUCED, RE-EDUCATES THE BODY!

exclusively devoted to this subject) we should touch bases generally with urine therapy generally and the wonders of our miraculous fresh urine. We swam in this for 9 months, fact no 1 and fact no 2 it was your mums pee first few months until you are a tiny little foetus self developed/formed a bladder then you swam in your own urine.

It was essential for you life form and who you are today, you drank it in the womb and also took it in through your nose, and it is now recognized that this amniotic fluid comprimised largely of your mums/your urine and is essential to grow the organs and lungs of your body.

Why Is Humanity rejecting fresh urine and urine therapy when this substance was what made us? We live in an upside down world my friend. Everything they tell us is a lie. Especially regarding health. It must be that way so we can be dependant on people outside ourselves (doctors!) To fix us and pills to pop to give us band aid solutions.

But these do not solve the root cause. Big pharma and pills never do. *The answer lies inside you.* Your own urine fresh from the tap is very powerful, it was designed as an instant medicine to clean out your pipe system, remove inorganic encumbrances that cause blockages and disease, to heal wounds cuts and bruises, to stop heart attacks and strokes, to save your life if you were stung by a poisonous animal even (hold under tongue your fresh urine twenty seconds after being bitten).

This all sounds so radical. Wasn't I brought up from birth with people telling me urine is a waste product. Didn't momma always tell me to wash my hands after going for a pee. They did. But they all been lied to. This is why this book is key. Fresh urine therapy is a good place to dive into true health and wealth, but there is enough information on this subject . *Aged urine is next level medicine. The key saviour of humanity.* So with that being said let us re-visit it as I plug deeper into its history (recommended by the Buddha!) and exactly why its so goddamn powerful. As I write this im 2 years into *Aged Urine*

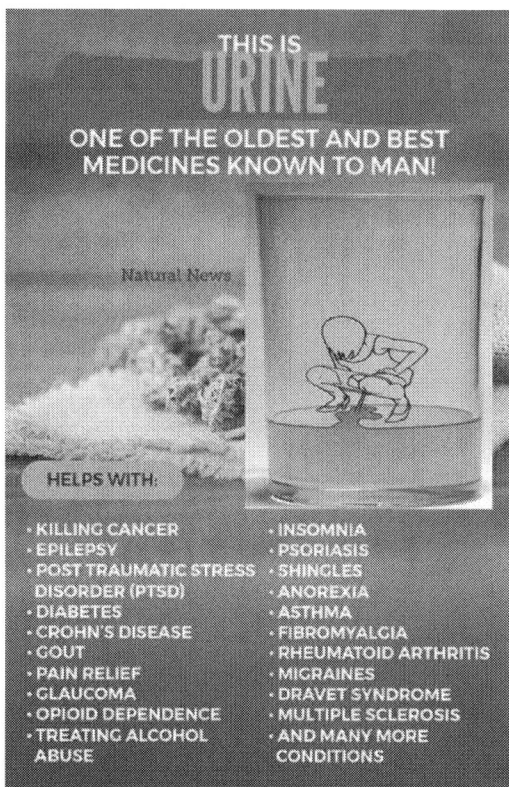

THIS IS
URINE
ONE OF THE OLDEST AND BEST MEDICINES KNOWN TO MAN!

Natural News

HELPS WITH:

- KILLING CANCER
- EPILEPSY
- POST TRAUMATIC STRESS DISORDER (PTSD)
- DIABETES
- CROHN'S DISEASE
- GOUT
- PAIN RELIEF
- GLAUCOMA
- OPIOID DEPENDENCE
- TREATING ALCOHOL ABUSE
- INSOMNIA
- PSORIASIS
- SHINGLES
- ANOREXIA
- ASTHMA
- FIBROMYALGIA
- RHEUMATOID ARTHRITIS
- MIGRAINES
- DRAVET SYNDROME
- MULTIPLE SCLEROSIS
- AND MANY MORE CONDITIONS

Therapy, long may that continue.

"The Virtues Of Human Urine, As A Medicine, Would Require An Entire Volume For Their Enumeration."-Sir Robert Doyle, 17th Century Pioneer in chemistry

Why Is Aged Urine So Goddamn Powerful! (the science stuff).

Negative Ions. Fresh urine is structured, all humans so long as we have breath in us are structured beings and our ultra filtered blood plasma(our fresh urine) is no exception. As it comes out it has a structure, leaving it negatively charged, making the urine perfect for re-ingestion back into our system as a negatively charged vessel to pull positively charged toxic crap out. *Heavy metals, excess* *mucus, inorganic crystals* and other such waste that usually get lodged in and take up space within our body leading to diseased states can be removed with fresh urine therapy, and the negatively charge contained within. Opposites attract, its pure magnetism and fresh urine has that magnetic charge.

But here's the key difference between fresh urine and aged urine. **The negative ion count grows** as the urine ages, more negative ions not only that but a smaller clusterization of the negative ions leading to an overall increase in the negative charge.

Think of it like this. Fresh urine and structured water found in fruits is a weak negatively charged magnet that pulls positive ion crap from your body. As the urine gets older and older it becomes a stronger and stronger magnet with vastly more pulling power as a consequence and aged urine will plug u deeper into happiness and health as a consequence of its ability as a strong magnet to pull more crap out.

Aged urine is a free medicine powerful enough with its strong magnetism to pull out decades and decades worth of filth from our colon(aged urine enemas), from our fascia and muscles (aged urine massaging) and brain (aged urine up the nostrum).

This was/is the one thing I missed out in my first book that I have since discovered as the main reason why aged urine is so powerful. As the urine keeps ageing and getting older, what was once fresh urine structured water becomes *aged urine uber super structured water.* There becomes no limit to just how structured the aged urine gets. Its negative ion count keeps on proliferating and getting bigger, but also the ever increasing negative ions get more compact and put into smaller clusters, thus rendering the existing negative ions more effective and increasing the magnetism of this powerful magnet exponentially. A stronger magnet pulls more. It gets more crap out. I say no more.

And all those who experiment with aged urine know it really does pull a lot of old ancient crap out of our system. The rising alkalinity of the aged urine(provable easy by any layman with a cheap pH meter of pH strips) maintains the structure of the aged urine as its stronger and stronger structurally, that magical *uber super structured water.* Gerald Pollock would so proud of our discovery! The 4th phase of water. There are so many crazy stories.

Aged Urine And Negative Ions

We have proved time and time again (and you can too by buying cheap ORP meter) that the amount of negative ions in the aged urine grows and grows with each passing day, and then not only that but the clusterization of these negative ions increases to smaller and smaller, making aged urine a *deadly weapon* for your health that will give you lots of energy, raise your vibration massively and send you into full on detox mode very quickly!

Negative ions alone are wondrous holy medicine that do many things, again all backed by science, like increase immunoglubin a (immune system function), increases movement of cilia, increase brain capacity, thinking speed and memory and provide extra oxygen for the blood calks and tissues. If you seek further information on negative ions please check out my book, *Negative Ions:The Grand Unifier Of Health And Life.*

Aged Urine And Nutrition.

All the ingredients present in fresh urine, all the vitamins, minerals, hormones, enzymes, neurotransmitters and stem cells are also present in your aged urine also , with a strong suggestion/ reason to believe that some of the magic in the fresh urine even proliferates, like the stem cells (science will confirm this one day for sure) and we already know the negative ion count increases, wow. Let me tell you that your aged urine is *the ultimate nutrition drink,* no nedd to buy expensive supplements when you got your aged urine.

How To 'Age' Urine

Like I did in my last book, to explain how to age is easy as simple as 1, 2 and Peeee. You pee in any bottle/container/mason jar glass or plastic, (preferably glass) and let the urine age all by itself. You can close the lid or leave it open to 'air' matters not to the ageing of urine. It does age slightly faster with open lid though if you want more power in shorter time. The urine is magical and it cant help but grow stronger and stronger as your *perfect medicine* with each passing hour and day. How amazing is that! By 4 days old your aged urine is quite strong, by one week very, by two weeks a deadly force of nature for your health happiness and vibration levels.

It has never been easier to be healthy and happy than with ageing yoke urine and then getting it into your system. I believe the future of mankind's health vibration lies with aged urine, and think of the costs in your healthcare once everybody knows and discovers this truth.

One day there will be emergency aged urine tanks and vats dotted around the road, the streets, the countryside everywhere for people in case of emergencies. This is the future PEEple.

To The Naysayers- Before You Dissent..

Before you voice opinions on this subject understand we have all been brainwashed from birth to believe urine as waste as a deliberate policy to subjugate man and keep under the whim of the doctor and medical allopathy and their beloved deities, the pills and drugs. When you understand this and

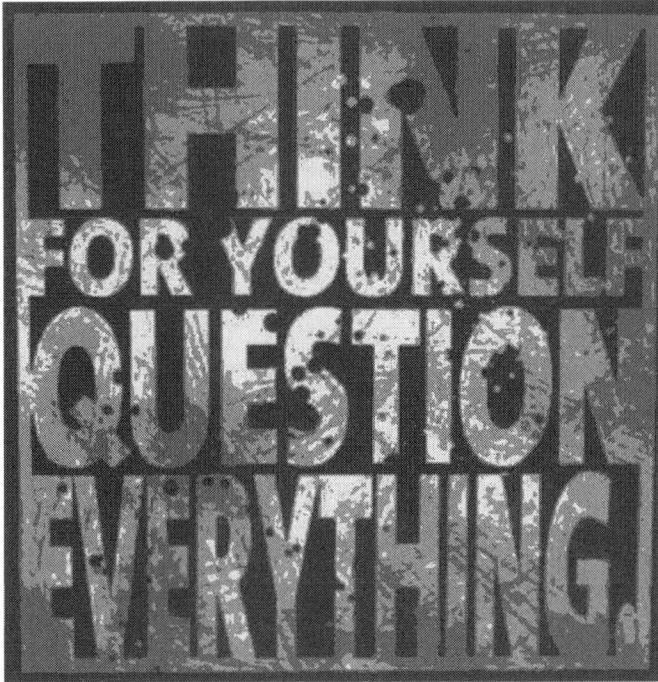

follow the rabbit hole of big pharma, the medical mafia, the real causes of disease, and the real cure, plus how our current healthcare system is absolutely destroying us as a species then u'll know or at least start to consider the possibility you were wrong.

Start questioning things. Always remain open minded. Do the research. Do the experiments. That's my biggest advice. You can conduct your own simple experiments with aged urine to prove that the thesis that it is a waste is a lie. Once you realize this you enter a rabbit hole if truth upon truth, seeing lie upon lie, you can never back away from, and it all begins with *urine therapy* and *aged urine*

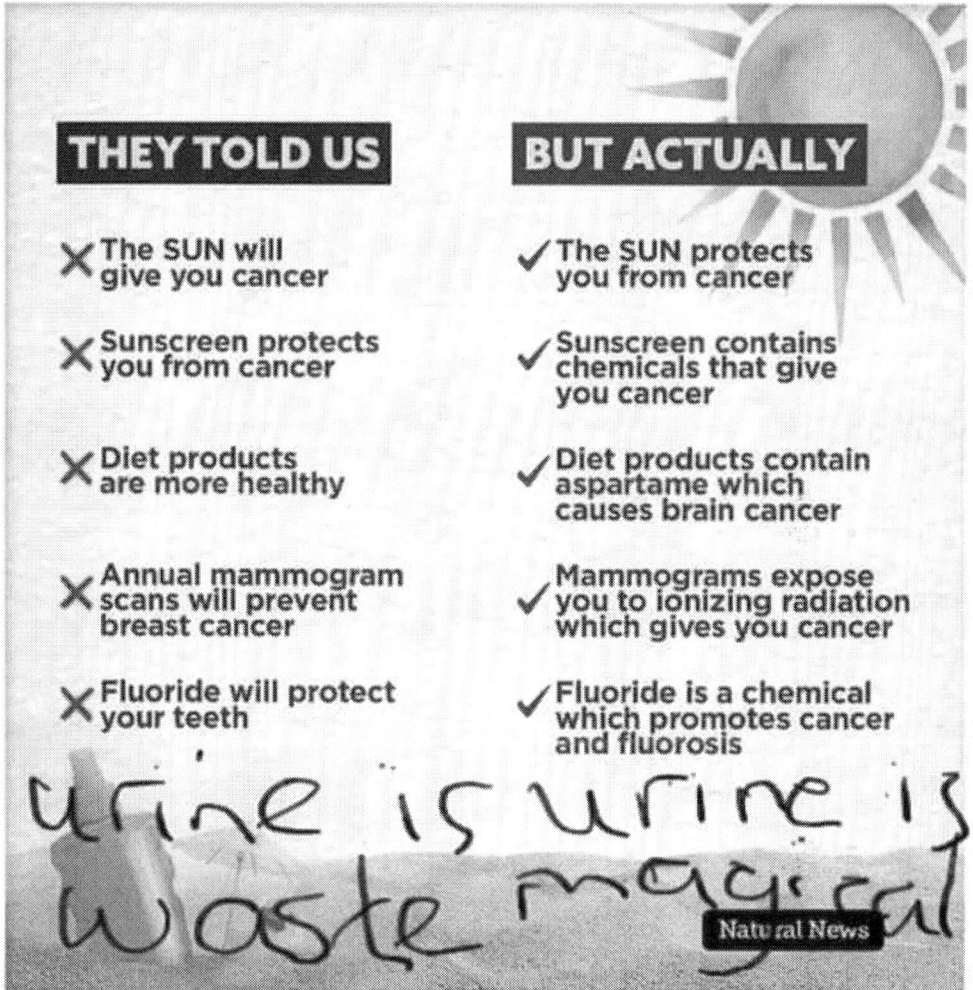

THEY TOLD US

✗ The SUN will give you cancer

✗ Sunscreen protects you from cancer

✗ Diet products are more healthy

✗ Annual mammogram scans will prevent breast cancer

✗ Fluoride will protect your teeth

BUT ACTUALLY

✓ The SUN protects you from cancer

✓ Sunscreen contains chemicals that give you cancer

✓ Diet products contain aspartame which causes brain cancer

✓ Mammograms expose you to ionizing radiation which gives you cancer

✓ Fluoride is a chemical which promotes cancer and fluorosis

urine is urine is waste magical

Natural News

Detox/Hexemeiner Reaction

When using aged urine expect severe reactions like feeling worse than before you took it, like nausea, vomiting, spots/acne coming up (with aged urine massaging) and headaches, lethargy/lack of energy etc. This is very common especially if we are new into health and detox and all it means is that the aged urine is *plugging deep* to heal you, pulling out a shit tonne of crap all at once, such is it's power to manifest health and raise your vibration levels. Not to be feared, this state is temporary, and once its out, its out! (Its actually a celebration when you get these reactions for that stuff that was hitherto previous inside can no longer stay stuck in body and cause harm and disease state. **Understand that aged urine is a very powerful healer of all diseases** and we will go into details into ways we could/should get it into our system to target different areas of the body and shore up our weaknesses.

You must get word before you get better, this is the rule of detox and hexemeiner.

Uber Super Structured Aged Urine And Water Viscosity

When a fluid becomes more structured, its viscosity changes. Viscosity is another fancy way of saying how smooth or stiff the water is. If its extremely viscous it means its very smooth and thin glides through the body much easier. Heavy stiff and thick water is less efficient never ideal and instead of cleansing your pipe work system of arteries veins and lymph it can even cause blockages. Can you guess how viscous aged urine is? Yep, its extremely thin smooth light and flowy, and fresh urine is too, but it gets more and viscous does the urine as it ages!

You will feel this viscerally (lol!) When you drink aged urine. It glides down the throat like you wouldn't believe. Try drinking tap water and bottled spring water. The difference in feel and viscosity between them is tremendous. Tap and bottled spring water with high ppm cause blockages within the body. They are heavy thick water full of inorganic minerals the body cant assimilate. All the nutrition in the fresh urine when aged is preserved by the ever rising *alkalinity,* which also preserves the uber super structuring process, Gerard Pollocks 4th phase of water (somebody ring Gerard Up, this is the one guys!)

This thin extremely viscous and smooth flowing Aged urine when it enters your system, this uber super structured water (uber super structured water is extremely viscous!) thins the blood instaneously, allows the red blood cells to hold into more oxygen, and more oxygen is transferred into the cells wow! This is where the deep slowed down breaths come from. From this process. Its a ginormous shift in consciousness. The extra oxygen assimilation into your system from taking Aged Urine can not be underestimated or over-exaggerated. Its huge! Plus every toxin that comes out of your body can only do so when bound to an oxygen molecule, and most people lack enough oxygen to detoxify their body properly, that is until you drink /imbibe aged urine or get in *any hole will do just get it in you!*

Less Breaths Per Minute On Aged Urine, The Key To Health

With extra oxygen in, and the body's increased capacity to utilize oxygen, we now have a lower metabolic rate and the body requires much less oxygen to thrive and function. We are holding onto more oxygen and not displacing it so quickly through too many breaths per minute.

A high breathing rate causes all kind of problems within your system including pH blood acidity, and all the various diseases which should come under one bracket and root cause. Shallow breathing and too little oxygen assimilation . *Slowing your breathing down and activating the para-sympathetic nervous system is one of the keys to health.* How to get there!? Get Aged urine into your system. For more info on this study up on Dr Buteyko's work.

Aged Urine And Your Sleep+ Dream Enhancement

Getting Aged Urine into Your system will majorly enhance your sleep function, pull you into ever deepening sleep, curtail the requirements of how long you even need to sleep, plus make your dreams vivid and you'll start remembering all your dreams again! How cool is that! One key reason we don't remember our dreams at night is we just don't focus on our health and sleep optimization, but Aged Urine will help majorly with that. It has me and many many others. One good to practice right before bed is to rub your Aged Urine from a spray bottle(Aged Urine Massaging) spray and rub it into forehead and temples. This practice will get the medicine right where its needed for great sleep and optimal dream recall, in your brain and pre -frontal cortex. The medicine seeps past the skull straight into brain! Also great to rub the temples with Aged urine before meditation or whenever you need extra willpower to do the right thing, again as the pre-frontal cortex willpower rational part of the brain holds the key here.

Aged Urine Is So powerful you will need less sleep and if you take it just before bed, drinking, enemas , massaging it in whatever way really you won't be able to sleep for a while. If this happens to you recognize its not a bad thing, like insomnia for example, but you are experiencing the bliss and high vibe state of the aged kicking in and lasting a long time.

Aged Urine And Depression.

Even fresh urine protocols work to relieve depression, they did for me anyway but the aged stuff is next level health vibration and the dark clouds become a thing of Christmas past. The brain often lies ruminate and tethered, its the brain and our thinking patterns that cause our poor vibration, but when we mess about with aged urine the brain calms down to its perfect natural state, like we were as a baby and child (remember all those happy childhood memories you had!).

Aged urine is so powerful a medicine as soon ad it hits the brain via the bloodstream there's a *massive shift in consciousness.* We know that depression in us is too much of high beta brainwave states which cause anxiety. Well what the Aged Urine does is it slows this high beta brainwave state right down to low beta and alpha wave flow state also, even theta, the doorway into the subconscious! This lifts the depression and parts the red seas and clouds of gunk holding us back. We feel so happy and ready to take on the world.

Aged Urine And Brainwave Coherence

Its not just brainwave speeds that cause depression mind. Also brainwave coherence. Which means how the brainwaves work together as one unit. An incoherent brainwave state leads to depression, anxiety, stuck in trauma, an inability to think properly and solve problems etc. The Aged Urine restores *coherence* to the brain such that each unit of the brain works more in harmony with each other. Its so bloody brilliant mate!

To extrapolate, think of coherence /incoherence as the difference between an orchestra with a conductor and one without. With a conductor the orchestra is led and guided to work in harmony with one another, without one there are problems not everyone is finding it easy to sing from the same song sheet (excuse the pun). *Aged Urine restores complete coherence to all parts of the brain,* and returns you to center point.

Aged Urine And Re-Balancing Of The Brain Hemispheres

Left brain right brain. Left brain is masculine in nature of the divine order, rational, logical, (overly critical lol),separate, ego driven. Necessary for our survival! right brain is feminine soft nurturing empathetic and one consciousness soul driven. We are all born into a matrix system that not only tells us huge *lies* like *urine is a waste product,* and that *looking at the sun will make us blind,* but also we are shipped out to school (prison) for many years of our life not only to brainwash us but to imbalance our brain hemispheres and keep us from accessing our divine nature which can only be accessed when our brain hemispheres are in balance.

Think about it. Why are we all forced to learn so much meaningless bullshit at school. It keeps us left brain.. Right brain is creative and soul work, schools do not encourage this. They beat out the personality and creation of every child. Now, not too go to far down this rabbit whole suffice to say:

Aged Urine definitely restores beautiful balance o the brain hemi-spheres, and not subtly either, you feel completely cantered within your body. Its so beautiful. Aged urine is so key to humanity taking its power back. To unleashing our creativity with a whole brain in perfect unison, to us becoming the best version of ourselves. If you haven't already tried aged urine, what are you waiting for? We are never really ready, just jump right in and experience it today. Experience is gnosis. (Know)(sis) and you'll know what im talking about.

Aged Urine And The Facebook Community

That's how I came to it. I read Martha Christy's book *Your Own Perfect Medicine* in a park in Birmingham in the summer of 2016, the rest is history. Tried it wow, dark clouds of depression I didn't know I had lifted. A new vibration for me. More than that was the excitement I could tap into this vibration readily again whenever I wanted at no cost due to my endless copious production of free medicine ushering forth as urine. I was so excited with the urine I went on to facebook search typed in urine therapy and found facebook groups that talked about it and joined them.

I learnt o much in those days. After a few months I had heard about *aged urine*, which I was hearing was even more powerful and the level up and natural progression from fresh urine. I had to try! And that was bliss. I became obsessed. More earning and more experiments continued. My vibration levels were through the roof. Too much energy. I talked so fast now my brain was running at mile a minute.

The facebook groups were tremendous help. I found real community of like minded souls there that wanted to help and share the knowledge of the power of aged urine. I started promoting it on my facebook wall. I started becoming known as the 'piss guy'. Didn't care. How could One? You're sitting on the most powerful therapies and healing modalities in the word. Aged Urine. Lets take a moment to be grateful and remind ourselves how lucky we are.

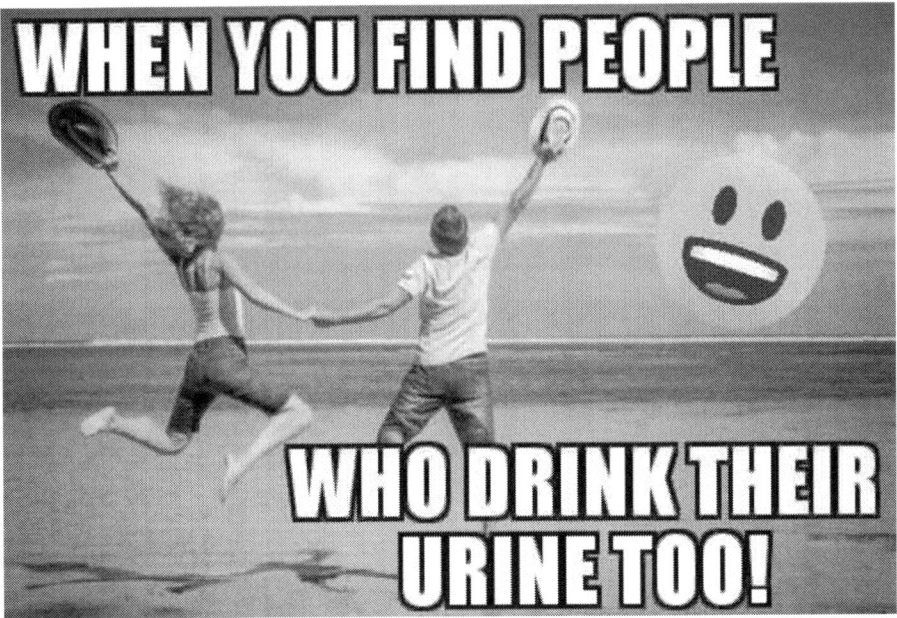

When you find people who drink their urine too!

We have a very active and growing facebook group on aged urine you guys can join for fee with a supportive community and people like myself as admin so join us there ask questions the meme below is the group to search for you can just type aged urine on facebook search also and find it that way. Namaste.

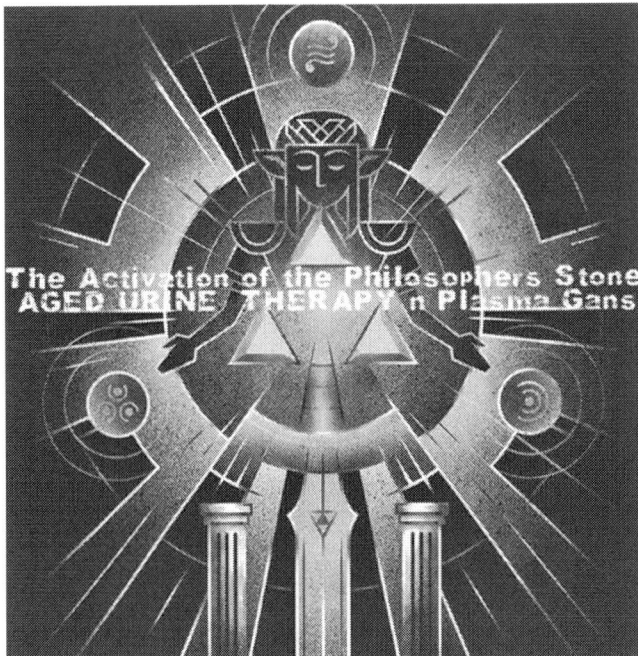

The Activation of the Philosophers Stone
AGED URINE THERAPY n Plasma Gans

I wrote my book on Aged Urine, the first ever exclusively devoted to this subject, in Jan 2019. It sold well and continues too today. I hope too write many more Aged urine books after this sequel in the future too, as new science comes in, we undo the programming and everyone's starts doing it (trust, in generations this practice will be completely normal!)

Aged Urine And Parasites

We all have them and this fact is undeniable. Some good , some bad. Most of us, the unhealthy have far too many, so one really powerful time and tested way to plug deep and remove the parasites hiding away in the small intestine and all over your body really is getting Aged urine into your system. Parasites are just like heavy metals and other toxic elements, they hold a strong positive charge. Anything that shouldn't be in your body and lowering your vibration like a parasite is positively charged.

We now know that aged urine is uber super structured water with a *very strong negative charge, a strong powerful magnet* that when confronted with a strongly charged positive ion parasite (they are really hard to get rid of with their strong magnetism) the aged urine washes them away and out of your system through the skin (aged urine massaging and yes, I've hears many a story of this!) or through the colon (aged urine enema's). Again I've heard many stories (myself included) of doing aged urine enemas and seeing parasite come out in the toilet, like tapeworms, roundworms large and small ones of funny colours.

 We are all infested with parasites to a varying degree, and they control our mood and vibrations. Have you ever felt 'hangry'? What is that? I mean you wont starve if you don't eat something every few hours. More often than not 'hangry' is the parasites inside you controlling your desire to eat and making you angry, to ensure you eat and ensure their survival.

3 powerful medicines that parasites actually hate. Dry fasting and Aged Urine and Turpentine!

Its not even the unhealthy generally that pull out parasite from deep within though. I've been part of the facbook urine therapy groups for 3 years now and some of the stories (and pictures!) Of parasites coming out the toilet after aged urine enemas is incredible. These parasites have been living in our gut hidden away there for many years and decades, some even stem back from childhood. *A pro-tip and one of the fastest ways to get them out is to do an aged urine enema in the dry fasted state, when you haven't eaten or drunk anything in a while, from 24 hours plus.*

Each parasite cleanse with aged urine removes blockages and vibration holds that stopped you accessing your best self. Each cleanse removes their control and power as they die off and realize the aged urine is too powerful. Its disgustingly beautiful lol.

Through the skin too. When we do the aged urine massaging its common to get a detox reaction of spot breakout on the surfaces of where we applied the aged, this is normal and very powerful, better they be out than in and cause diseases down the line. (that's how diseases work btw. Toxicity buried deeper and deeper within never given the opportunity to come out until a tipping point is reached where the body can no longer have the space to store the toxins and you get 'symptoms'. For me personally I know when parasites are coming out after I've massaged aged urine over my gut as my bum starts getting itchy and these are often very small microscopic ones the naked eye cant see even.

Along with spot breakouts with the aged urine massaging sometimes people report parasites coming out of the skin. Itchiness and then this thing. Seeing is believing in this case, watch and observe, the body never lies!

Pro-Tip- For ultimate parasite cleanse do aged urine enemas regularly plus aged urine massaging over gut daily.

AGED ORIN

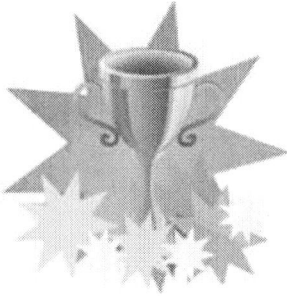

FOR

=

A

CLEAN COLON

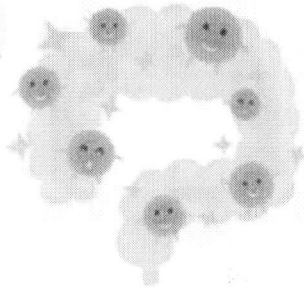

Aged Urine And Cancer

We know that fresh urine contains at least 7 anti cancer elements which include *HUD, H11 extract, Retine, Anti-neoplastons, Uric acid, Hydrogen Peroxide* but there will be many more discovered in the near future as we know our blood and body is always working for us and always fighting off cancer every single second and hour of every single day. Add high doses of negative ions and smaller clusters of Aged Urine combined with uber super structured water and hormones like *melatonin*(anti cancer hormone) you've got in Aged Urine one of the most potent anti cancer remedies on earth, all at your beck and call.

If you g ot specific cancers you can wisely target those organs areas with aged urine massaging as well as aged urine enemas and aged urine drinking, under the tongue, aged urine pulling etc. With diseases and cancers you want to go *all out* to fight it off give yourself the best possible chance disease free and aged urine will give you that chance so up the amounts of aged urine you use plus combine it with dry fasting . (Breaking dry fasts with aged urine protocols are the best!)

Aged Urine Darkens Your Skin

Wow cool, what does this mean? Is it a good thing or a bad thing. Well im with 20th century Legend Arnold Ehret on this one. When your skin gets darker (your version of darker) you are getting healthier and healthier and if your skin is getting paler you are getting weaker and sicker. This was one of the smartest observations ever made in my opinion.

Think what happens when you out and expose your skin to midday summer sun. You get a tan. A skin tan. A healthy glow. Your skin darkens for your protection and this darkened skin (your version) is a true indicator your getting healthier. But also when we drink aged urine, and especially when we massaged aged urine into skin, your skin darkens and bronzes most beautifully!

This darkened skin now indicates true health and that we are removing copious amounts of harmful excess mucus from the system, as Arnold Ehret stated and I am with him on this. *I love aged urine massaging and its ability to give you a natural tan,* its ultimate sun screen protection too to the 'harmful' uv b rays of a midday sun or any sun if you live in the tropics.

Aged Urine Massaging is the best suncream protection you will ever need atop the fact it makes your skin glow.

Think of people who go pale with shock or sun burn at the beach on holiday, go a pasty red colour like a lobster. This paleness of skin, and burning when confronted with the sun, indicates a truly unhealthy individual who is full of toxins and mucus, who will reap what they sow with ill health and maybe even early onset death. You cant be too careful these days. *Start today, with Aged Urine therapy!*

Aged Urine Warms The Body Up And Increases Circulation

As a result of getting aged urine into your system (any hole will do!) Your body warms up in an instant, its crazy to watch and experience this! Coldness internally is a poor circulation issue, in the same way those with diabetic neuropathy have coldness in the extremities due to poor circulation, and this sign of ill health can be remedied so easily with *Aged Urine Therapy*. The blood vessels start dilating and relaxing, blood flow to all parts of the body increase as soon as the aged stuff hits the circulatory system.. More oxygen is retained in the haemoglobin, which now travel single file with their strong negative charges and the blood thins out. This single file red blood cell strong negative charge aged urine action means the red blood cells can get into the tiniest and flimsiest of capillaries straight into the cell. Its the fine capillary networks that connect us to the cells for our cellular nutrition and waste extraction and sticky red blood cells cause blockages in the capillaries so cell extraction and nutrition becomes impossible.

Aged Urine Thins Your Blood

Thick lumpy blood is the cause of many a problem in your body when ideally we should all be healthy and have oue blood flowing around us like a smooth fine wine, extremely viscous. We already know aged urine is that smooth fine extremely viscous substance, so upon entry it goes to work thinning your existing blood out and delivering its magnetism to the waters and all the cells in your body.

Sticky thick blood leads to heart attacks, strokes, arthritis and you name it all the diseases under the sun so when you make your blood thin and smooth flowing, no blockages can present themselves, and the negative charge power magnet of the age goes to work pulling out all the toxic crap (positive charges) within my system.

Thin Smooth Flowing Blood for the win, thank you Aged Urine!

Aged Urine Massaging For Women. Look 10 Years Younger..

Not even kidding. The fresh urine you produce and capture already has 2. 5 % urea, which is a top world class moisturizing agent used in the best anti skin ageing products, but when the urine ages, its uber super structuring effect and increased smoothness and viscosity allows for it to make skin glow and shimmy like you just couldn't imagine.

This experiment is easy to try. Store your fresh urine in a plastic or glass spray bottle let it sit and age for a couple of weeks then spray on your face. Watch as you de-age yourself. Your face will appear much younger and well bronzed too, this is the power of aged urine massaging it in.

Aged Urine Massaging is ine of the topways t get aged urine into yoyr system, not to mention fine looking ddope ass skin. De-age yourself today, with Aged Urine.

Beauty is only skin deep they say. Well Aged Urine massaging is the way! Its the secret of the supermodels their youth and dope ass skin. Urine therapy and particularly Aged Urine Massaging. What women wouldn't want to look twenty years young at 30! To maintain that youthful glow and attractiveness long past when they should! Welcome initiates, start with aged urine massaging today!

Aged Urine Massaging feels like the perfect pee coat protection, and holds you to your highest state of vibration, less easily triggered, more the real you, impervious to any situation.

Aged Urine And Quality And Quantity Of Life

Aged urine protocols regularly committed too will affect both. You wont be seeing the inside of a doctors office or a hospital anytime soon if at all, the quality of your health and happiness will improve, and most probably u'll give live alot longer than if you hadnt discovered and used this powerful medicine.

You are blessed indeed my friend. Imagine too the mind-set and belief that using Aged Urine Therapy will give you. That you are all powerful. That your body has its own self healing mechanism. That you have free potently powerful free medicine.

Aged Urine Drinking And Firewater

When you drink your Aged urine as we recommend, you'll notice a heavy kick and you won't be able to drink too much all in one go. We call it the firewater. Continue sipping it in small amounts this firewater is not harming you (aged urine never does!). My theory as to why it has such kick to drink is that there is a proliferation of hydrogen peroxide in your ageing urine. Why? Because of our cooked foods and wrong eating, the fresh urine produces white blood cells to combat. A by-product of the white blood cells fighting with the foods we ate is hydrogen peroxide. So in fresh urine the white blood cells and hydrogen peroxide are in small amounts but as the urine ages the white blood cells proliferate in number to deal with the cooked dead food we gave them and create more and more hydrogen peroxide (H202). Its the growing amount of hydrogen peroxide I feel that makes aged urine the firewater. This is not a problem. Hydrogen peroxide is good for you and safe in the aged urine. Please drink it.

Another proof to me of my proliferating white blood cell/hydrogen peroxide theory is the fact when you eat pure fruits for example or fast, those aged urines captured have no kick, no firewater is created at all. They are easier to drink. This would be because the white blood cells do not recognize the fruits as a poison and they didn't proliferate and need to generate hydrogen peroxide as their by-product. Its a fascinating thing to think about and I hope we can prove my theory correct in the near future. We know also uv light and blue sunlight (midday suns) triggers increased white blood cell count and more hydrogen peroxide, could this be one reason why aged urine ages quicker with solarisation?

For now note that your aged urine contains high amounts of hydrogen peroxide, which is a healthy protocol to do in and of itself, so aged urine is like hydrogen peroxide therapy plus more some!

Aged Urine And Pro-Biotics

As well as being ultimate supplement drink, aged urine is very special as the ageing process proliferates all the beneficial bacteria which when reingested populate your gut microbiome with a huge amount of beneficial good bacteria. The aged urine as it ages each passing day increases its amount of these pro-biotics which feed the good bacteria and make more of them wow!

Nowadays pro-biotic supplements and pro-biotic drinks are getting hugely popular as science catches up to the mechanisms of its power to heal the body and gut. It all makes sense! And as Hippocrates the father on modern medicine once said *"all diseases begin in the gut".* The gut is like your second brain and when you heal all kinds of magic happens and diseases clear away. The organs of the body start firing optimally its beautiful to watch and witness. To feel alive inside your body. Aged urine's pro-biotic factor feeds and multiplies the good bacteria whilst its uber super structuring high negative ion strong magnetic effect eliminate more and more of the parasites and harmful bad bacteria. Bad bacteria in the gut also cause depression, anxiety and low mood. By getting aged urine into the gut you tackle this problem head on. I cant think of anything more amazing right now, no other medicine quite like the aged urine.

Aged Urine And Magnetism

Our health relies upon strong magnetism. For we human beings are magnetic and electric. The negative ions are electric and re-supply your body with tremendous electricity for every cell to work properly, and this uber super structuring effect of aged urine leaves it as mentioned earlier with a *very strong negative charge,* it becomes a very powerful magnet. The magnetism of aged urine is off the charts and leaves it liable to pull toxins, heavy metals and parasites from deep within your system. Remember, *Aged Urine is extremely magnetic and electric.* When your body vessell loses its magnetism and electric power, diseases can creep into the poison environment and overwhelm you.

Aged Urine and Breathwork

Breath work is such a huge facet of the high vibe life and optimal health, slowing the breath down, but here's the thing. Drinking Aged Urine or getting it into your blodstream any other way really (under the tongue, massaging into skin, enema's) is the breath work. It causes a profound shift in consciousness and slows the breath down major in an instant which lasts for up to 24 hours. Therefore getting aged urine is your breath work. And slowing the breath down is the key to optimal health, vitality, energy and living a long time free of diseases and other encumbrances.

You can of course do breath work daily on top of aged urine protocols as I do to optimize but make sure *Aged Urine is your foundational daily health protocol go to for the most powerful as your daily priorities* .

Aged Urine And Your Metabolism

Metabolic rate /metabolism means quite simply the rate at which you consume oxygen. Those who are unhealthy and diseased state have a high *resting* metabolic rate, and are consuming a lot of oxygen just to stay alive. In fact the high resting metabolism is what's causing their il health! But what Aged Urine does is pretty special. It supplies your entire vessell with more oxygen , makes the tissues alkaline, so they can now hold on to more oxygen, and *lowers your metabolic rate.*

Aged Urine increases your oxygen capacity and use /assimilation of oxygen drastically such that your resting metabolic function is now much less, your body's requirements of oxygen go down, less is more, and you thrive with abundant energy supplies.

Key takeaway: The Lower your metabolic rate the longer you will live and the healthier/energetic you will be, and Aged Urine slows the breath down and does just that, it lowers metabolic function. A huge ant-ageing weapon.

Other Ways Not Mentioned In First Book To Get Aged Urine Into Your System.

Big one. Vaping. Vaporisation of the Aged Urine. Go on amazon buy a cheap Vaporization machine (mine cost £40 and had tonnes of good reviews) and start vaping the urine today! This is one of the most powerful ways to get the Aged in. It turns the liquid Aged into a gaseous element which is then breathed into lungs, where it becomes a highly penetrating weapon of health clearing out the finest elements of toxic substances in your lungs and also clearing out the mucus from the key breathing areas super fast. It shocked me when I did, how much better I breathed after vaping aged urine and breathing it in in gas form wow! And you use do little urine too. Only a few drops produces a helleva lot of gaseous aged for vaping!

If you have COPD, Asthma, or any breathing diseases or diffuculties, maintain a good Aged urine protocol , but focusing especially on vaping aged urine will be most beneficial and give you the fastest results. Whenever we mess about with aged urine the results are tremendous! Also vaporizing the urine uses very little of it, it makes it most efficient, a bit like Aged Urine Massaging.

Another really good one is taking Aged Urine baths, pouring what Aged Urine you have saved away there in your bathtub , where it will be diluted but is such powerful medicine it works a holy wonder. I've done it before and no one notices there's no smell even and the rising hot tub heat means you get the fumes of the medicine into your system as well as it seeping into your naked skin all over. Wonderful!

Aged Urine Is Like Red Light Therapy, But Way Way More Powerful.

Well thats a bold statement. But no exaggeration. I love sunrise /sunset red light therapy, ever since I got into it in in May of 2019 I woke up at sunrise every day outside or windows open the red light bathing my naked skin. Its very powerful for sure, red light being to me the most important colour of the sun, hence the red light therapy machines we have nowadays, but to say Aged Urine is a notch above even this form of concentrated sunlight is fair when you expedience both of them. Sunrise Subset bathing your eyes and skin that one is a subtle shift up that gives us abundant energy depending how long of sunrise/sunset we stay out for, but just a few dips of a few weeks old aged urine, is a *major not so subtle shift in consciousness.* Interestingly, both red lght therapy and aged urine work by similar mechanisms...

Aged Urine Is More Powerful A Healing Modality Than Sunlight Even.

Aged Urine Is Jet Fuel For Your Mitochondria

As soon as this uber super structured fluid gets into the cells and the mitochondria which fuels the cell the Nano motor of the krebs cycle process ATP production gets enhanced and speed up *majorly* thus providing the sufficient fuel for the mitochondria to ramp up its ATP production and provide us with extreme amounts of energy. Its crazy until you experience it. *Jet fuel for the mitochondria.* And however you get Aged urine into your system matters not as all cells in and around where aged is applied get the good stuff, the fuel, and we'll talk about later how aged urine is *localized* and *systemic* medicine which you may find interesting. The Aged urine and red light therapy give the mitochondria oxygen for increased ATP production (the aged urine more so even) but also this kicks out nitric oxide from the mitochondria and into the blood circulatory vessell walls causing a *major dilation of your entire blood and capillary networks.* This blood vessel dilation slows the breath down and gives us extra energy removing blockages and allowing the body to work more freely.

The Damar Tantra And How The Ancients Knew About The Power Of Our Urine.

This is an ancient text written in India centuries before Christ BC on how urine made one feel magical and blissful and outlined what this medicine would do to the individual if they went on a prolonged period of urine therapy. Instead of explaining it I thought why not better than go straight to soyrce and post up some memes of a direct translation of it. It is copied on the next few pages please take the time to read it.

URINE IS BETTER THAN ANY DRUG FROM A DOCTOR

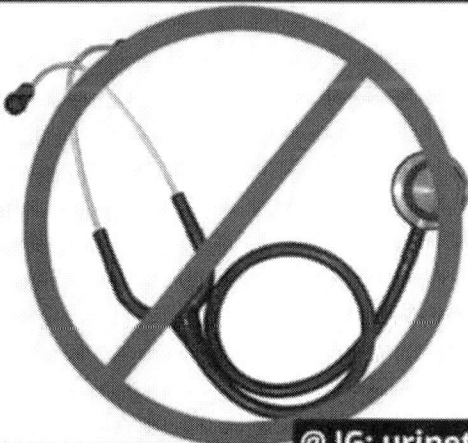

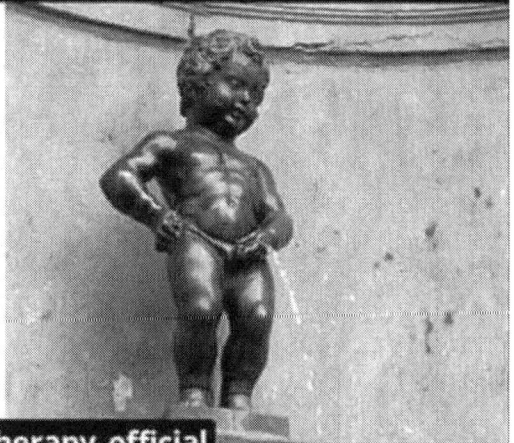

@ IG: urinetherapy_official

Regularly it is said that, "if urine is so good how come doctors don't prescribe it?" they don't because they are NOT ALLOWED to by their elite, W.H.O. In the 19th c. doctors experimented a lot with many substances in desperation for cure to many diseases, one of these notorious experiments was with URINE. It was they, the doctors, who coined the term 'urine therapy'. They would collect urine from public bathrooms and use it to test on various diseases and infecting organisms (DESTROYING the diseases with urine), this was how urine was established as 'anti-cancer' and 'anti-viral'! The history speaks for itself. But because they could not loot money off the public with Urine Therapy, they condemned it as "waste", this is why you hear it being called that everywhere. So, urine is historically and has repeatedly been experimentally proven to be the BEST MEDICINE your body NEEDS.

Auto-Urine Therapy (Shivambu Kalpa):
The Indian version as detailed in the DAMAR TANTRA.

O Parvati! I shall expound to you the recommended actions and rituals of Shivambu Kalpa that confers numerous benefits. Those well versed in the scriptures have carefully specified certain vessels for the purpose. (1)

Utensils made from the following materials are recommended: Gold, Silver, Copper, Bronze, Brass, Iron, Clay, Ivory, Glass, Wood from sacred trees, Bones, Leather and Leaves. (2, 3)

The Shivambu (one's own urine) should be collected in a utensil made of any of these materials. Among them, clay utensils are better, copper are by far the best. (4)

The intending practitioner of the therapy should abjure salty or bitter foods, should not over-exert himself, should take a light meal in the evening, should sleep on the ground, and should control and master his senses. (5)

The sagacious practitioner should get up when three quarters of the night have elapsed, and should pass urine while facing the east. (6)

The wise one should leave out the first and the last portions of the urine, and collect only the middle portion. This is considered the best procedure. (7)

Just as there is poison in the mouth and the tail of the serpent, O Parvati, it is even so in the case of the flow of Shivambu. (8)

Shivambu (auto- urine) is heavenly nectar, which is capable of destroying senility and diseases. The practitioner of Yoga should take it before proceeding with his other rituals. (9)

After cleansing the mouth, and performing the other essential morning functions, one should drink one's own clear urine, which is the annihilator of senility and diseases. (10)

One who drinks Shivambu for the duration of a month will be purified internally. Drinking it for two months stimulates and energizes the senses. (11)

Drinking it for three months destroys all diseases and frees one from all troubles. By drinking it for five months, one acquires divine vision and freedom from all diseases. (12)

Continuation of the practice for six months makes the practitioner highly intelligent and proficient in the scriptures, and if the duration is seven months, the practitioner acquires extraordinary strength. (13)

If the practice is continued for eight months, one acquires a permanent glow like that of gold, and if it is continued for nine months, one is freed from tuberculosis and leprosy. (14)

Ten months of this practice makes one a veritable treasury of luster. Eleven months of it would purify all the organs of the body. (15)

A man who has continued the practice for a year becomes the equal of the sun in radiance. He who has continued for two years conquers the element Earth. (16)

If the practice is continued for three years, one conquers the element of Water, and if it is continued for four years, the element Light is also conquered. (17)

He who continues the practice for five years conquers the element Air, and he who continues it for seven years conquers pride. (18)

Continuation of the practice for eight years enables one to conquer all the important elements of Nature, and continuation of it for nine years frees one from the cycle of birth and death. (19)

One who has continued the practice for ten years can fly through the air without effort. One who has continued it for eleven years is able to hear the voice of his sour (inner self). (20)

He who has continued the practice for twelve years will live so long as the moon and the stars last. He is not troubled by dangerous animals such as snakes, and no poisons can kill him. He cannot be consumed by fire, and can float on water just like wood. (21)

O Goddess! I shall tell you now about other variants of the therapy. Please listen attentively. He who takes powdered *amrita* (*gaduchi*, Tinospora Condifolia) mixed with Auto-Urine habitually for six months, is freed from all disorders, and acquires happiness. (22, 23 cont...)

Powdered *haritaki* (*harade*, Terminalia Chebula) should be assiduously taken with Shivambu. This combination destroys senile degeneration and all diseases. If this practice is continued for a year, it makes one exceptionally strong. (...23, 24)

One *masha* (about one gramme) of sulpher be taken along with Shivambu every morning. He who continues the practice for three years will live as long as the moon and the stars last. His urine and feces will whiten gold. (25)

The powder of the *Koshtha* fruit should be mixed properly with Shivambu and taken in the prescribed manner. If this practice is continued for twelve years, one's body will be free from the ravages of old age such as wrinkles on the skin, and whitening of the hair. One acquires the strength of a thousand elephants, and lives as long as the moon and the stars continue to exist. (26)

If powdered pepper and *Triphala Choorna* (mixed powder of Terminalia Belavica, Terminalia Chebul and Phylonthus Embica) mixed with Shivambu are taken regularly, one acquired a radiance like that of the gods. (27)

The essence *(bhasma)* of mica and sulpher should be taken with Shivambu along with a little water. This cures al disorders caused by malfunctioning of the digestive system and all disorders caused by the *Vata* humour. He who takes such a mixture regularly become strong, acquires a divine radiance, and can cheat time (escape the ravages of time). (28, 29)

He who takes Shivambu daily and excluded salty, sour and bitter food from his diet acquires divine accomplishments quickly. Freed from all ailments, and possessing a body comparable to that of Shiva Himself, he disports himself like the gods in the Universe for an eternity. (30).

Aged Urine Re-Discovery Of The Century Recommended By The Buddha Himself

There are found in the *Pali Canon* the early buddha texts four mentions of **aged urine** as a medicine the buddha himself recommended to his initiates to be healthy and be enlightened even. Its my belief also that the buddha did not find enlightenment alone from his vipassana meditation and keeping his posture still for very long periods of time. The key piece to getting to that stage of enlightenment was his assiduous use of *aged urine* and why he recommended his followers use it. He was aware of its power to amplify the vessell and raise your vibrations and consciousness level, not to mention he was happy to share and promote for all a wonderful *free* healing modality. Let us now explore his quotes.

The Buddha, The Pali Canon And Aged Urine

The original texts were in Sanskrit also so lets translate and find out what the buddha was referring to and meant. In Sanskrit :-

Puti=fermented.

Mutta=Urine.

Bhesajja=Medicine

Putimuttabhesajja=Fermented Urine As Medicine

Though some comentators explained the Pali expression putimuttabhesajja to mean fermented cows urine, nowhere is the word cow (govi or go) mentioned in the original texts. Others have explained the word 'puti' to mean "that which is repulsive" and implied that the Buddha recommended fresh urine therapy-drinking one's own fresh urine "although it is repulsive". But Puti clearly means fermented, putrid, decomposing. For instance the word 'corpse' in Pali is puti kaya, that is a rotten, decomposing body. What follows are *quotes of the buddha from the Pali canon, the standard collection of early Buddhist scriptures.*

"Putimuttabhesajjam nissaya pabbajja tattha te yavajivam ussaho karaniyo"

Going Forth has fermented urine medicine as its support. For the rest of your life you are to endeavour at that.   Mv.1.77.1T

Note:-"going forth" means becoming a buddhist monk or nun. The Buddha taught his monastic disciples to use fermented (aged) urine as their go-to medicine!

"Medicants, these four trifles are easy to get hold of and are blameless. What four? Rag -robes, a lump of alms-food. Lodgings of the root of a tree. **Fermented urine as medicine.**   Anguttara Nikaya 4.27

"These four, bhikkhu's, are trifling things easily obtained and blameless. What four? A robe made of cast-off rags is a trifling thing, easily obtained and blameless. Food gathered as alms is a trifling thing, easily obtained and blameless. The root of a tree as a dwelling place is a trifling thing, easily obtained and blameless. **Medicine consisting of putrid urine** is a trifling thing, easily obtained and blameless. These Bhikku's, are the four trifling things, easily obtained and blameless. When a Bhikku is content with these things, that are trifling and easily obtained, I say of him that he has the requisites of recluseship.

-seem to a householder or a householder's child 10

Note:- 'Bhikku's' means beggars/recluses/monks and nuns, monastic disciples of the buddha.

"As you live contented your **fermented urine as medicine** will seem to you like various medicines-ghee, butter, oil , honey molasses and salt- seem to a householder or a householders child. **It will be for your enjoyment, relief and comfort, and to reach Nirvana.**   Angutarra Nikaya 8.30

I love this verse from the buddha particularly because it goes upon his usual assertions that aged urine should be the go to medicine but also states its a way to reach Nirvana/Enlightenment and I fully agree with him, its very very powerful medicine!

"Now at that time a certain monk had jaundice. 'I allow you, monks, **to make him drink aged urine** and yellow my robalon.   Theravada Vinaya Pitaka Khandaka Mahovagga-6.

Note:- In Theravadan countries to this day aged urine is known as the Buddha's medicine.

"Suppose there was some fermented urine mixed with different medicines. Then a man with jaundice would come along. They'd say to him. 'Here, mister, this is fermented urine mixed with different medicines. Drink it if you like. If you drink it the colour, aroma and flavour will be unappetizing, but after drinking it you will be happy.' He wouldn't reject it. After thinking, he'd drink it. The colour, aroma and flavour would be unappetizing but after drinking it he would be happy.   Majjhima Nikaya 46

*"Anyone who makes use of leftovers for food. **Putrid Urine as medicine,** the root of a tree as lodgings. And rags from the rubbish heap as robes, Is at home, In any direction.*   Theragatha 18.1

It seems obvious to me from these buddha quotes and my own direct experiences with aged urine, and those of many others around the world and on facebook groups, that aged urine is powerful medicine designed for us to heal ourselves from anything and take us to our highest vibration.

Aged Urine And Pharmaceuticals.

This is a key topic and area of concern for many people. We do know that pharmaceutical drugs we take do come out in the fresh urine unfortunately. But here's the thing. A truth that will shock people. As the urine ages and grows in *alkalinity,* the ageing urine completely nullifies and neutralizes any toxic pharmaceutical that were originally present in it.

Let me repeat that again. As the urine ages, it completely nullifies and neutralizes all pharmaceutical residues. And toxins. And heavy metals. And anything detrimental to our health present it all gets taken away, neutralized. Wow! This is ground-breaking phenomenal news! After about two weeks there is zero residue of anything negative in the aged urine, what's left only is the preservation and proliferation of the good stuff. This is huge.

All the naysayers concerned with toxins coming out in their pee, when they fast or due to their toxic consumption need not worry as aged urine completely neutralizes everything bad. If you put enough cyanide to kill someone in it for example by two weeks that aged urine would no longer present with any trace of the stuff and u'd live (don't experiment on humans though!). As of present we in the urine therapy community are not suree why he aged urine does this by which process, it might be the ever rising alkalinity (pharma drugs are acid) or the uber super structuring extreme negative charge which pulls all inorganic crap (positive charges!)in the body. I look forward to science investigating what im saying here sometime in the future as its easily provable in their labs with a couple of simple experiments. In the meantime we are the scientists of today and tomorrow so don't fear, we experiment and bring you the best info!

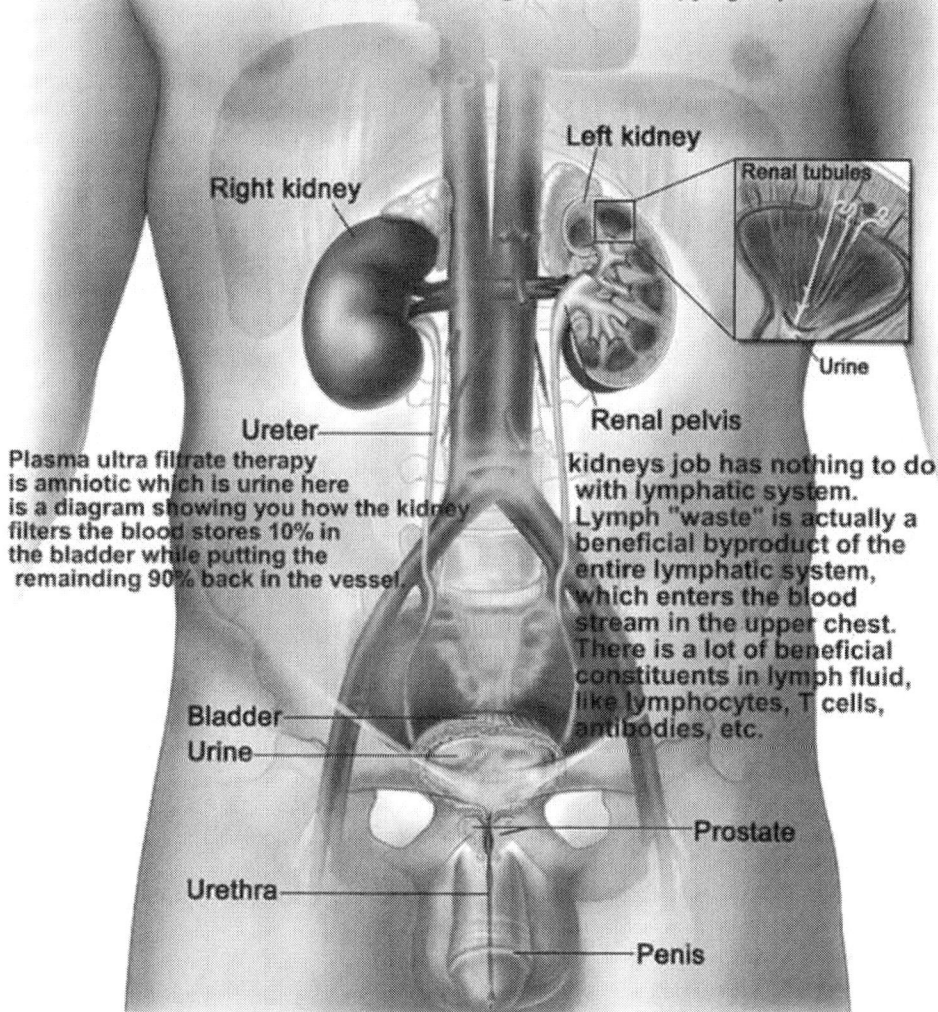

Left kidney

Right kidney

Renal tubules

Urine

Ureter

Renal pelvis

Plasma ultra filtrate therapy is amniotic which is urine here is a diagram showing you how the kidney filters the blood stores 10% in the bladder while putting the remainding 90% back in the vessel.

kidneys job has nothing to do with lymphatic system. Lymph "waste" is actually a beneficial byproduct of the entire lymphatic system, which enters the blood stream in the upper chest. There is a lot of beneficial constituents in lymph fluid, like lymphocytes, T cells, antibodies, etc.

Bladder
Urine

Prostate

Urethra

Penis

Aged Urine And Stem Cells

Science has however admitted and investigated that there is indeed stem cells present in all of our *fresh urine.* So our aged urine has them too! But we also suspect that not only does the aged urine contain the stem cells present in the fresh, but the *stem cells actually proliferate and grow in number* as the urine ages. We believe this because people report miraculous healing of wounds with aged urine, and whiles these could be explained a little by uber super structuring effect of aged urine and high negative ion count (negative ions heal wounds) the stem cells factor cannot be underplayed and just overall there's a strong suspicion that the stem cell count grows and grows in our aged urine. For me personally im 32 now and for the past two years of me being on Aged Urine therapy I have been getting 'growing pains' in my legs, the pains I used to get as a teenager when I was at my biggest growth spurts. The fact I'm still getting them now @32 and only during periods after aged urine consumption tells me all I need to know. The high ever growing stem cells are making me grow taller at a time according to 'science' when I should have stopped growing lol.

Fresh Urine has Stem Cells And Aged Urine Proliferates the Stem Cell Count. No need for expensive stem cell treatment just get on Aged Urine!

Aged Urine Neti Pot Cleansing

This is a great one and another way to get it in. The Hatha Yoga Pradipika states that "neti pot cleanses the cranium and bestows clairvoyance. It also destroys all diseases above the throat". I concur, and especially when you use one of the most powerful medicines on earth, aged urine in your neti pot. The nose, eyes, inner ears and brain will get cleansed and using this as part of a daily routine, the neti pot aged urine, will transform your health, slow the breath down, increase oxygen uptake and allow for optimal health. Instead of people showering in dirty unfiltered tapwater and brushing their teeth with fluoridated toothpaste every day they should be doing aged urine net pot (if you do the opposite of what the unhealthy masses do you will be more than likely healthy and funny how they think urine is waste product). NOTE :- Aged urine neti pot will burn your inner face off and the mucus will pour out the nostrums, so be warned, and recognize this is not a bad thing. Its wiping the crap off and re-generating tissue in there. The old adage 'no pain no gain' is true for many aged urine protocols like aged urine in eyes and up the bum in enemas also.

Whichever way you choose to use Aged Urine just get it in you, any hole will do! Choose multiple holes even. Up the nose. Up the bum. Massaging it into skin. Under the tongue.

Aged Urine Oil Pulling And Swishing

For great oral hygiene this one is great to experiment and witness crazy results. Get some aged in mouth don't swallow though instead swish it around and around like you do those mouthwashes. The aged urine will pull all the toxic crap and harmful microbes/bacteria in your mouth and transform the mouth microbiome to a much healthier one which will improve your overall health overall and have you feeling great. I highly recommend this one daily along with brushing your teeth with Aged Urine (is there anything aged urine can't do?..nope, not in my experience!)

Note:- If you have mercury fillings do not do this one, please have them removed first, as the aged urine will sit there and pull the mercury out and into gut, contaminating your body with extra toxicity).

Aged Urine The Ultimate Shampoo And Conditioner

Just want to throw it out there. Aged urine on your hair seems to make the hair glow and shine just like the skin! So so beautiful. Not to mention it seeps into cranium healing the brain also. It makes a great hair gel for men, a conditioner of hair for men and women when left in there, and a brilliant shampoo you can apply all over and rinse out. Many people report this and I have heard so many testimonials on facebook groups to know this truth. Try it and see yourself!

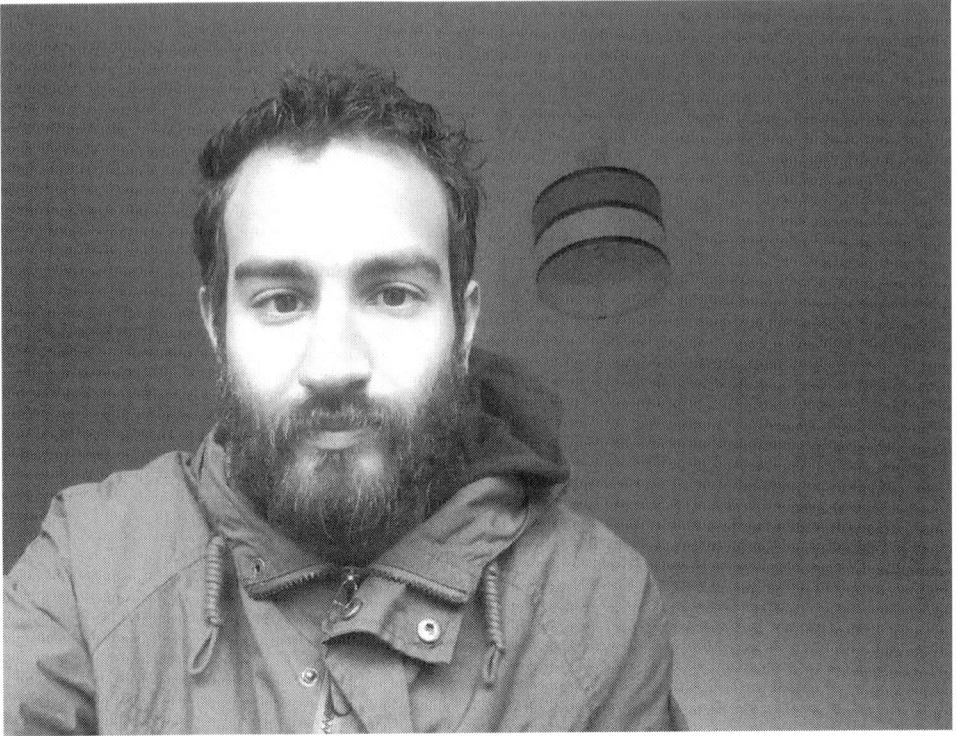

(The author a photo of after aged urine massaging onto face his daily protocol plus massaging into hair using it as shampoo conditioner and hair gel). God bless Shivambu!

Aged Urine Massaging Onto Testicles For Gentlemen

This is a simple routine for guys that will transform your health happiness and vitality. Massaging Aged urine over your sexual chamber will majorly increase sperm production and majorly ramp up production of all important hormone called *testosterone*. Testosterone is such a key hormone for guys to have a lot of I cant emphasize this enough. Many men now are suffering from endemic low testosterone levels with takes away their happiness ad health, takes away not just their sex drive but their ambitions, fearlessness and creativity too. Testosterone is a success hormone in guys as much as a happiness and health one, high testosterone allows men to achieve the impossible! It gives you fuel and motivation.

One of the best ways to have high testosterone levels is to start massaging aged urine over your testicles on a daily basis.

Check out my youtube videos I made on this key topic you'll find them on my channel @holistic health with harry or even if you just typed aged urine testicular massage on the YouTube search bar. I'm pioneering this stuff and know it works because I feel it uber charging my testosterone levels especially if its a few weeks old aged urine as that aged urine grows in potency and a few weeks old is very powerful.

Aged Urine Massaging Over Yoni For Women

A women's sacred sexual chambers benefit from massaging aged urine over it just as much as men. Her oestrogen levels will optimize to crazy high levels and her testosterone levels (women need testosterone too!) will stabilize making her feel crazy good and crazy powerful happiness and health are not exclusive , they are intertwined , and when a women massages her aged urine onto her sexual parts she will experience bliss not to mention as well make her eggs as pure as they can be and increase chances of fertility same as the man increases his chance of fertility and creating a baby with aged urine massaging over testicles! Wow

In both men and women, the sacred sexual chambers make the key sex hormones of oestrogen and testosterone, and the key to their optimization and proper function is aged urine massaging over yoni and testicles.

For Geeks. Best Time To Get Aged Urine In!

Anytime is a good time for Aged urine really. That's what I tell people new to this stuff. You want to experience the magic first before geeking out with amplifying your vessell further by getting the habits nailed. As a rule, *the emptier your tummy (fasted state) when you take the agped urine in, by whatever means, the better and the more powerfully it will deliver results.*

For example, if you dropped an a ged urine enema twenty hours of not eating any food at this time expect better results than dropping one 4 hours after having eaten food. Same with drinking it or any other way. The emptier your tummy the better. Aged Urine protocols are a great strategy to mitigate the damage done by eating cooked foods and junk food too, which one will experience but should not use an excuse to carry on maintaining an improper diet without improvement.

If one did an aged urine enema deep into a fast except to see much mucoid plaque, worms and parasites in the toilet. This medicine is so powerful and when combined with fasting it becomes super super potent the parasites cant handle that purity and seek an early exit from your bowels sometimes from having been there from your childhood.

Aged Urine pulls layers of deep toxicity from the body. When in the fasted state, even more so. Ultimate magnet.

Aged Urine And Fasting

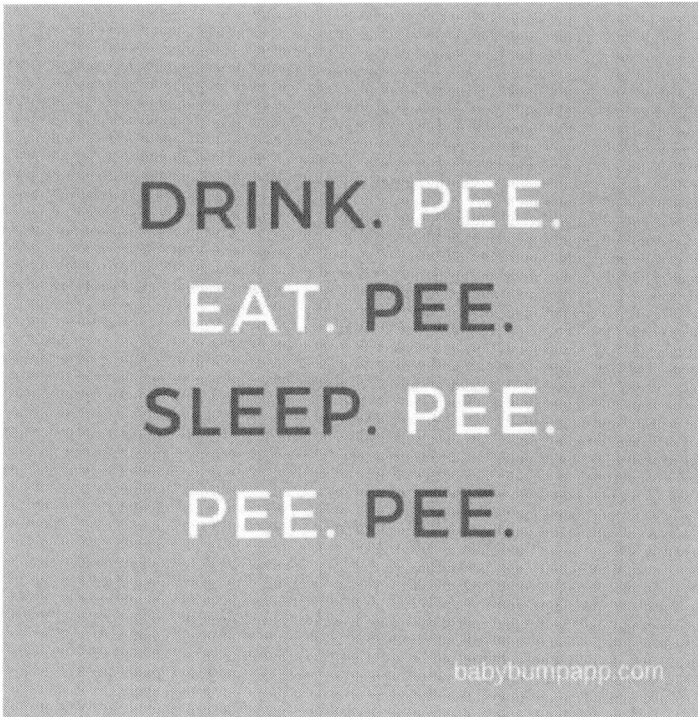

DRINK. PEE.
EAT. PEE.
SLEEP. PEE.
PEE. PEE.

babybumpapp.com

Aged Urine combines really well with fasting. Definitely recommend and a great way to break a fast too by drinking it or dong an Aged Urine enema. During fasts one can do any Aged Urine protocols to amplify the detox process and clear the junk out the trunk faster, and something like aged urine massaging whole body rubs in the fasted state speeds up everything and helps your body pull toxins out at this key time.

Aged Urine Drinking Vs Aged Urine Massaging.

Both extremely powerful but I wanted to specify that some of the magic of ages urine is lost when drinking it compared to when we massage it on the skin. It could be that in drinking it the stomach acids destroy the sensitive hormones in the aged urine or some of the aged urines alkalinity is lost in the stomach with the hydrochloric acid, making Aged urine massaging one of the most powerful ways to get all that nutrition and uber super structured water in with nothing lost. Direct shot into o bloodstream and cells.

Aged Urine Massaging Is Localised And Systemic Medicine.

Drinking Aged Urine or under the tongue action is also different to massaging in that it only delivers you systemic medicine. What this means is the medicine gets all around the body via the blood/circulatory system targeting everything but in small amounts. You cant pick and choose an organ or a part of the body to go all out in with the medicine with systemic medicine only. Its still goad, but here's where Aged urine massaging comes in as extra special.

Aged Urine Massaging is also systemic medicine, but also localized too! When you rub your aged urine say over your liver, the medicine will be localized and seep right into the liver itself as well as also being systemic as the skin is fulll of blood so the aged urine makes its way all around the bkdy via the blood /circulatory system too! This makes aged urine doubly powerful, not to mention how little of the aged urine is actually used massaging it its a win win !

You can target specific ailments and problems, like weak adrenals/kidneys, liver , colon, thyroid, weak legs etc with the aged urine massaging and getting this systemic and localized medicine in, plus no loss of power by going through the digestive system and straight into the bloodstream which lies only 1/ 10th of a millimetre below the skin surface (prick your skin with pin you will see if you don't believe me).

Currently I'm doing some aged urine massaging in morning first thing upon awakening at sunrise time and last thing before I go to bed at night for approx 10 minutes each. Let me tell you a little goes a long way with this small amount of aged urine use, it comes highly recommended as one of the most efficient and best uses of our holy shivambu medicine.

You will notice your aged urine smells, but that's not a problem if you drink it, up the bum in enemas, under the tongue etc, only presents a challenge with aged urine massaging so strategies around this include doing them massages last thing at night as the smell goes away completely after only a few hours, plus using essential oils on skin after, and also massaging fresh urine over the skin after (latter point takes away 70% of trace smell). You can stack them too, doing all 3. No smell is key so as not to ostracize yourself and offend people. Stay safe fam.

Which Fresh Urines Are Best To Capture For Our Aged Urine

Simple answer. It doesn't really matter. I want you if you're just starting out to capture any fresh urines, not just the oft talked about first of the morning mid streams, but any really. Why? Because as the urine becomes aged, even in the most unhealthy of people, it becomes holy powerful. J W Armstrong found this out in the 1930's and 1940's when he healed thousands of sick and dieing people with their own aged urine, massaging it in for 1 hour plus (the longer you spend here obviously the better). I highly recommend peope read his book, *The Water Of Life,* which has re-popularised this therapy to western nations along with *Martha Christy's* excellent *Your Own Perfect Medicine.* For current times I have a dear brother called Dave Phillips who has written another excellent one, combining the powers of Urine therapy with eating only meal a day, essentially a fasting +urine diet, called *OMAD ORIN LOOPER,* I have re-read it several times and i hope you re-read mine!

For the geeks and hard-core mad scientists the best urines to capture for ageing are first of the mornings when you're in fasted state naturally, after you have just eaten something good for you and nutritionally sound, like fresh fruits and vegetables, and the best of the best, the cream of the crop is the *fasting urines,* those ones captured deep into a fast, be that a juice fast, a water/urine fast, and especially a *dry fast (*future book on dry fasting inbound at some point, its along with aged urine the top two of healing modalities).

Urines captured in this pure state make very special aged urines that will amplify the vessel in super quick time. But to repeat, all aged urines are holy, mighty and worthy. Try it and see! (don't even believe me).

How To Speed Up Your Aging Of Urine

For the geeks in the house I guess. Who want to heal. from diseases faster. Who want to optimize the vessell as quickly as possible. Firstly *solarisation* aka leaving your urine bottle to age outside in sunlight, especially the sunrise and sunset red light therapy suns. All sunlight frequencies structure the urines quicker, but especially visible and invisible red frequencies of sunlight. So leave it out under (cloud cover) sun.

No 2. As mentioned in my first book, the urine will age with lid open or closed. However a closed lid does indeed slow down the ageing process so with that being said, if you can, open the lid or put a breathable cloth over, to speed up its ageing!

Thirdly you can use the power of magnetism by putting your urine bottles over a magnetic water coaster for example. The stronger the magnet the better. This structures the ageing urine even faster than if you did not use it, i experience this speeded up more powerful aged urine every time i leave my urine to age over a magnetic water coaster and this is further proof to me my theory that the main mechanism of power of aged urine is its *uber super structurization* its stronger magnetic effect. The alkalinity of the aged urine maintains that structure. So bottom line, use strong magnets or use a magnetic water coaster.

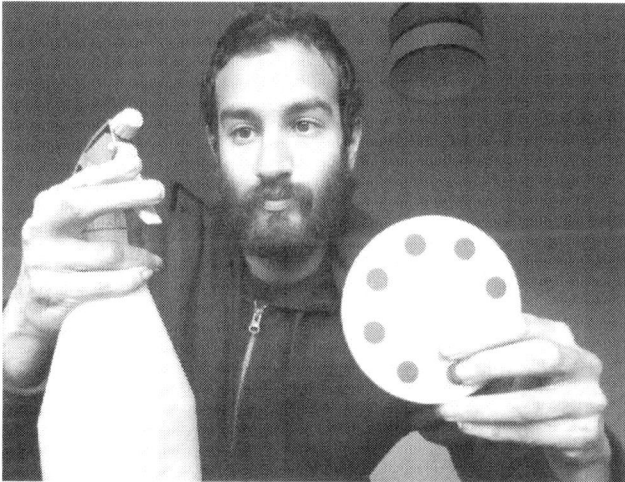

Aged Urine An Electricity And Magnetism

Aged urine is extremely electric and highly magnetic. Its deep electric energy run through the size cluster and sheer quantity of negative ions plus uber duper super structured super viscous (smooth/fine) water allows our body to recieve the electricity it needs to function to its highest potential.

The deep magnetism of the aged urine runs in there pulling up the deepest set/stuck of patasites, toxins and heavy metals because these are all positively charged. What do opposites do? Attract! There's no need to complicate the wonders of aged urine too much as these are definitely the main reasons why its more powerful than sun. And don't forget, aged urine preserves the nutrients hormones, enzymes, neurotransmitters (serotonin dopamine GABA etc),making it the ultimate supplement drink.

Conclusion

If you want more information see ,my youtube channel where I have many aged urine videos., you can find them @holistic health with harry, also add me on facebook @harrymatadeen as my handle, where I also talk and share about it.

The tips are out there too for free. Buy my first book on aged urine too, for a how too on the myriad powerful wats to get aged urine into your system. And our aged urine group on fscbook, where we have a strong community of like minded souls on your journey into aged urine and urine therapy

Lastly I would like to leave you with a message to enjoy life make the most and not take it too seriously.. yYour aged urine will transform your health vibrancy and level of consciousness but never forget our life here in duality is temporary so lets all be silly! Namaste. Harry

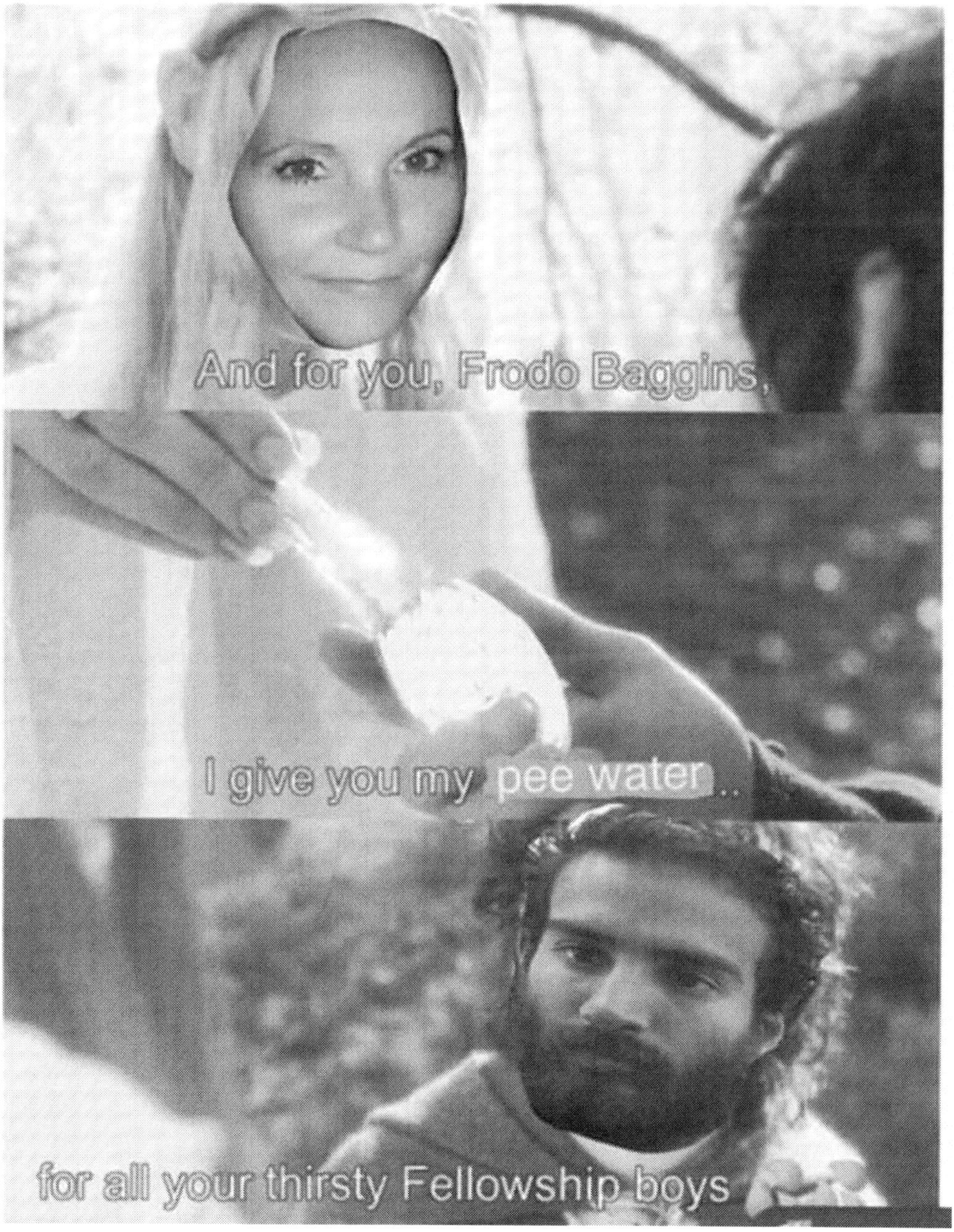
And for you, Frodo Baggins,
I give you my pee water..
for all your thirsty Fellowship boys

You want "spirituality"

Mantras

Crystals

Soul mates

And twin flames

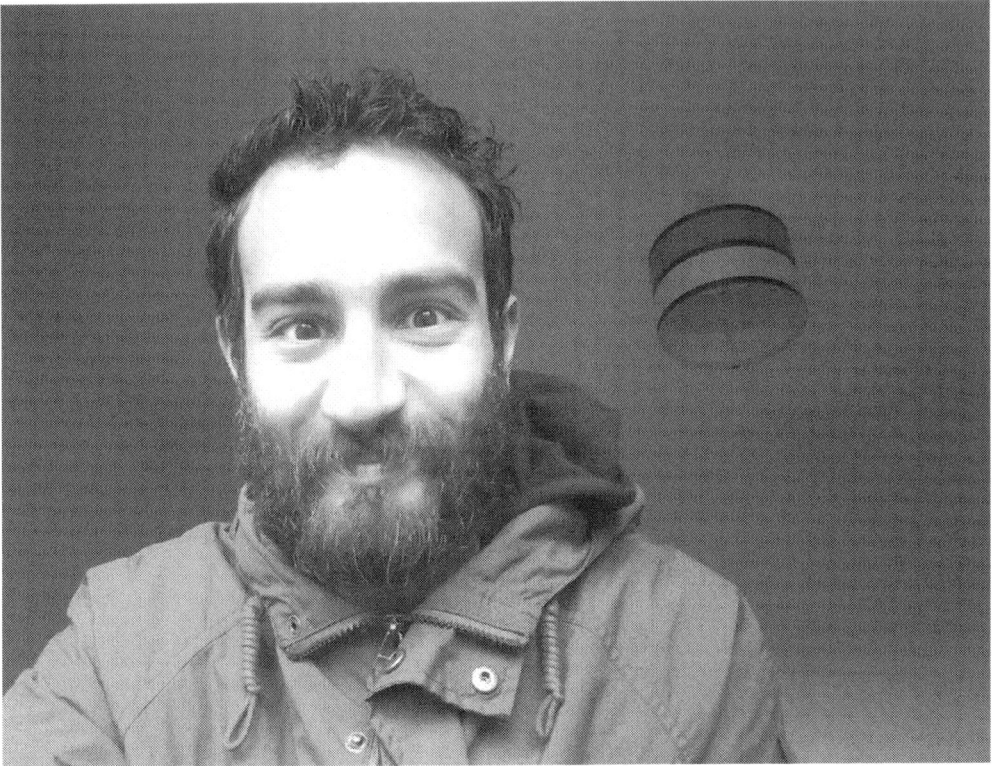

You want

The perfected state

The unperturbed

Presence and

 love

But do you want truth?

Real truth

Truth borne

> APPRECIATION
> IS THE PUREST
> VIBRATION THAT
> EXISTS ON THE
> PLANET TODAY.
> —ABRAHAM HICKS

Of brokenness

Truth

That you finally see

When you hit

The lowest of the low.

Or is your spirituality

Another costume

That you are wearing

To be someone

To make sense

To be accepted

Loved

Respected

Needed?

I can't help

But sense

That this search

We are all on

In the name

Of spirituality

Is just a clever way

To avoid

Having our hearts

So broken open

That the very dirt

Beneath our feet

Becomes

Holy.

We fear the pain

Of this breaking

So much.

How could it be

That the darkest

Or most mundane parts

Of our existence

Are also breathtakingly

Exquisite?

How could it be

That our memories

Our bodies

Our relationships

Our lack of meaning

Our addictions

Our patterns of sabotage

Are actually divine jewels?

SOMETIMES IT TAKES AN OVERWHELMING BREAKDOWN TO HAVE AN UNDENIABLE BREAKTHROUGH.

The sheer divinity

Of reality

Just as it is

Is so overwhelming

For the mind

That the concepts

Of "spirituality"

We create

And so loyally follow

Become another shield

Of protection.

Better to drop down

To the lowest point

Naked of all pretence

Completely defeated

Unable to adhere to

Any form of spirituality

And then just wait

Until your eyes

Open up.

If there is such a thing

As "spirituality"

This is it.

~James Marshall

HEALTH BENEFITS OF TEARS

Like the ocean, tears are salt water. Protectively they lubricate your eyes, remove irritants, reduce stress hormones, & they contain antibodies that fight pathogenic microbes. Our bodies produce three kinds of tears reflex, continuous, & emotional.

Each kind has different healing roles. Reflex tears allow your eyes to clear out noxious particles when they're irritated by smoke or exhaust. The second kind, continuous tears, are produced regularly to keep our eyes lubricated— these contain a chemical called "lysozyme" which functions as an anti-bacterial & protects our eyes from infection. Tears also travel to the nose through the tear duct to keep the nose moist & bacteria free. Typically, after crying, our breathing, & heart rate decrease, & we enter into a calmer biological & emotional state.

Emotional tears have special health benefits. Reflex tears are 98% water, where.as emotional tears also contain stress hormones which get excreted from the body through crying. Emotional tears shed these hormones & other toxins which accumulate during stress. Crying also stimulates the production of endorphins, (our body's natural pain killer) & "feel~good" hormones." Humans are the only creatures known to shed emotional tears, & maybe elephants & gorillas do too.

Crying makes us feel better, even when a problem persists. In addition to physical detoxification, emotional tears heal the heart. You don't want to hold tears back. Whenever i cry i get embarr3ssed or worried my energy is effecting someone else & i try to suppress the tears. It makes me feel weak. I know where that sentiment comes from~parents who were uncomfortable around tears, a society that tells us we're weak for crying. I reject these notions. Try to let go of untrue, conceptions about crying. It is good to cry. It is healthy to cry. This helps to emotionally clear sadness & stress. Crying is also essential to resolve grief, when waves of tears come over us after we experience a loss.

Tears help us process the loss so we can keep living with open hearts. Otherwise, we are a set up for depression if we suppress these feelings. There is nothing to apologize for.

Let your tears flow to purify stress and negativity.

When we suppress our tears, we suppress our healing.

THE BENEFITS OF CRYING

- It activates the parasympathetic nervous system aka our calm state
- It releases toxins from the body
- It releases stress hormones from the body
- It releases oxytocin and endorphins, which help to relieve pain and elevate mood

Charlie Chaplin Poem

As I began to love myself

I found that anguish and emotional suffering

are only warning signs that I was living

against my own truth.

Today, I know, this is Authenticity.

As I began to love myself

I understood how much it can offend somebody

if I try to force my desires on this person,

even though I knew the time was not right

and the person was not ready for it,

and even though this person was me.

Today I call this Respect.

As I began to love myself

I stopped craving for a different life,

and I could see that everything

that surrounded me

was inviting me to grow.

Today I call this Maturity.

As I began to love myself

I understood that at any circumstance,

I am in the right place at the right time,

and everything happens at the exactly right moment.

So I could be calm.

Today I call this Self-Confidence.

As I began to love myself

I quit stealing my own time,

and I stopped designing huge projects

for the future.

Today, I only do what brings me joy and happiness,

things I love to do and that make my heart cheer,

and I do them in my own way

and in my own rhythm.

Today I call this Simplicity.

As I began to love myself

I freed myself of anything

that is no good for my health –

food, people, things, situations,

and everything that drew me down

and away from myself.

At first I called this attitude a healthy egoism.

Today I know it is Love of Oneself.

As I began to love myself

I quit trying to always be right,

and ever since

I was wrong less of the time.

Today I discovered that is Modesty.

As I began to love myself

I refused to go on living in the past

and worrying about the future.

Now, I only live for the moment,

where everything is happening.

Today I live each day,

day by day,

and I call it Fulfillment.

As I began to love myself

I recognized

that my mind can disturb me

and it can make me sick.

But as I connected it to my heart,

my mind became a valuable ally.

Today I call this connection Wisdom of the Heart.

We no longer need to fear arguments,

confrontations or any kind of problems

with ourselves or others.

Even stars collide,

and out of their crashing, new worlds are born.

Today I know: This is Life!

Charlie Chaplin

Water runs a river

Through the body it flows

Mother always told me; we reap what we sow

And so the water of life Eye drink

My truest cellf ,the missing link

Every answer to every question

Inside me all along

When listening carefully eye can hear the song...

The rhythm of my heart and all the codes within

Emerging to the surface, healing my ancestral kin

Looping e fountain; body on the mend

Shivambu; the greatest teacher

Pure light, our divine god send

An alkaline avatar; our natural state to be

It's never been so easy, u need only to drink your wee

OMfessions of a pee drinker

-
-
-

#vegan #rawvegan #fruitarian #frugivore #rawfoods #alkaline
#urinetherapy #shivambu #orintherapy #looping #structuredwater
#barefoot #grounding #earthing #recycle #healing #detoxification
#rejuvination #homeostasis #parasitecleanse #muciodplaque

Jess sie

WHY and HOW is aged urine more powerful thank fresh urine?

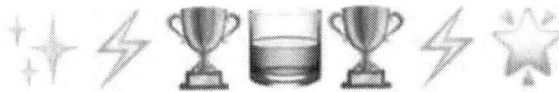

✨ ⚡ 🏆 🥃 🏆 ⚡ ⭐

A Post By Monica Schutt On Why Aged Urine Over Fresh.

WHY AGED URINE A POST BY Changa Charanga

I feel the inner impulse to address some misconceptions about AGED URINE... I hope you don't mind my involvement in the discussion or "debate" in this way... but it is so much I have to say, that it would be more fair to share it as a new post instead of packing it in a comment section. :)

⚠️ FIRST MISCONCEPTION I FIND is when people say aged urine is only for "external" use....:

🙆 When we apply aged urine on our skin, we are also "drinking" it through our pores. It is an "external" use, but it is actually an INTERNAL TAKE, as powerfully healing as it would be introducing the aged urine through the mouth or any other way.

⚠️ SECOND MISCONCEPTION I FIND is when people think it is "too powerful" to start with, that it's better to start with fresh urine only....:

🙆 There's no reason to fear the power of our urine. When it's aged, it enhances its power simply because it has had time away from the unhealthy habits we subject our bodies to on a daily basis - which of course affect the purity of its water - and so the urine as it is held in a new container that is not the body, has the chance to work on its own purification... PERFECTING ITSELF... becoming a much purer medium to hold the light of divine spirit, so it reaches a HIGHER VIBRATION, thanks to "fasting" and if we use THAT *high vibrating (aged) urine, we will get much more LIGHT into our bodies, much more HELP of this DIVINE ENERGY! ✨ ✨ ✨

This can only do us GOOD!!

Why fear it?

There's absolutely no reason to fear this LIGHT - it's DIVINITY itself. It can only do us good and it will never be a shock or anything bad for our system. Only our fears are all that. But not love... and this energy is PURE LOVE.

This divine energy - or perfect LOVE - KNOWS how to act best in every situation and under any circumstance... for every body, for every person, so it will not create any shock or unnecessary experience. WE CAN ALWAYS FULLY TRUST IT and surrender to its action... IT'S a SUPREME DIVINE LOVE, that CARES PERFECTLY FOR US, BEYOND ANYTHING WE CAN IMAGINE....!
🫣😊🧎✨👃👅💫

And I find it totally understandable that the people who have experienced this powerful love, this amazing divine care - thanks to their own use of aged urine - will want to talk about it and share with others very passionately.

⚠️ THIRD AND FINAL MISCONCEPTION I FIND is that aged urine consumption do not belong into the UT practice because there is no literature on it...:

🦉 Aged urine is part of the urine therapy as it is plain URINE... simply in a much purer state... and books are written thanks to the new experiences people have made, right? It's thanks to the "pioneers" that books about certain practices or modalities started to exist and we all have this pioneering spirit in us, which allows us to grow and evolve... share in books/ written, it also furthered the development of literature and humanity... so, why should we stop or put our pioneering spirit ever on hold?

There's no reason not to continue making more new discoveries and experiences just because we haven't read about them in books about... what kind of reasoning would be to live our lives only based on pre-existing knowledge we found in books? To only base our life experiences on what's been written by others in a book? Do we really think we so limited and incapable of something else, something more? What about our own book :D ? I know each one of you has their own book written in your soul and I WOULD ACTUALLY LOVE TO READ THAT BOOK!!! I know it's awesome!! A real best seller!! Only not yet printed out.

Our own soul teaches us all truths... and it is not limited to any external literature.

Also our ancestors knew so many of these truths and many were passed unto us through word of mouth only... or perhaps they were as well written in all the books which had been burned, among all of the real knowledge that the "wanna be controllers of this world" tried to silence and continue to attempt their censorship!

Let's not fall into this category of people wanting to control or limit our real expansion, to stop or hinder our own exploration to reach full awareness. All truths are found within, not limited to external books, but primarily in our own book.

If I don't see any books on a certain subject or no words in the pre-existing books dedicated to a subject of my interest and study, which of course (as with all things) can always be DEVELOPED FURTHER, then I find only MORE REASONS and encouragement to investigate further beyond what the pages of those books show me, through connecting with my own inner soul guidance and following its impulses, making my own experiences, doing my own exploration and discovery... then naturally SHARING MY FINDINGS WITH ALL the people who are interested, and I think THAT'S WHAT GROUPS ARE FOR... so we can all continue growing through our interaction, sharing our testimonials, exchanging our findings and views... this to me is making/ writing more books in the flesh and never stop or settling for anything other than the full discovery of ourselves in this fantastic opportunity of our life existence... I only wish for us all to keep on learning & growing like that... pretty much free style, only paying attention to stay within the natural frames of love and respect.

I love all UT groups and I'm truly very grateful for all the work and dedication admins and members put into them, to keep the groups alive... they are for me a wonderful and sacred ground, a perfect support system, much needed to inspire and strengthen our ever continuous growth...! ✨ 😊 🍃 ✴️

I TRULY THANK YOU Monica L. Swift AND ALL IN HERE FOR ALL YOU DO!!! I know it's all done with the best of intentions and so is this text I'm now sharing...

Printed in Great Britain
by Amazon